2012 Drug Information Update

Drug
Information
Update

for
Davis's Drug Guide for Nurses, TWELFTH EDITION
and **Nurse's Med Deck,** TWELFTH EDITION

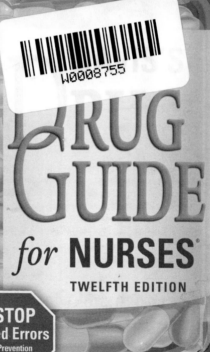

W0008755

DRUG
GUIDE
for **NURSES**
TWELFTH EDITION

**STOP
Med Errors**
Prevention
Strategies

Judith Hopfer Deglin
April Hazard Vallerand
Cynthia A. Sanoski

Drug Updates - www.DrugGuide.com

Judith Hopfer Deglin, PharmD
Consultant Pharmacist
Hospice of Southeastern Connecticut
Uncasville, Connecticut

April Hazard Vallerand, PhD, RN, FAAN
Wayne State University
College of Nursing
Detroit, Michigan

Cynthia A. Sanoski, BS, PharmD, FCCP, BCPS
Chair, Department of Pharmacy Practice
Thomas Jefferson University
Jefferson School of Pharmacy
Philadelphia, Pennsylvania

ISBN 10: 0-8036-2312-7
ISBN 13: 978-0-8036-2312-5
Printed in the United States of America.

Note: As new scientific information becomes available through basic and clinical research, recommended treatments and drug therapies undergo changes. The author(s) and publisher have done everything possible to make this information accurate, up to date, and in accord with accepted standards at the time of posting. The authors, editors, and publisher are not responsible for errors or omissions or for consequences from application of the information, and make no warranty, expressed or implied, in regard to the contents of the information. Any practice described in this information should be applied by the reader in accordance with professional standards of care used in regard to the unique circumstances that may apply in each situation. The reader is advised always to check product information (package inserts) for changes and new information regarding dose and contraindications before administering any drug. Caution is especially urged when using new or infrequently ordered drugs.

2012 DRUG INFORMATION UPDATE

The **2012 Drug Information Update** presents the full pharmacologic profile for 48 newly approved drugs and is for use by those who have purchased **Davis's Drug Guide for Nurses, 12th Edition** and **Nurse's Med Deck, 12th Edition**. Designed for portability, the update may be inserted inside the *Davis's Drug Guide* for Nurses or used with the *Nurse's Med Deck*. This supplement in addition to our postings on www.DrugGuide.com will completely update the current editions of *Davis's Drug Guide* and *Nurse's Med Deck*. Having this Update available precludes the need to purchase another 2011–2012 drug reference and thereby offers you substantial savings.

Keep up-to-date at www.DrugGuide.com

Gain free access to new drug monographs, the latest FDA approvals, innovative articles on pharmacology, drug alerts, dangerous side effects, and potentially life threatening drug-drug, drug-natural product, and drug-food interactions.

Contents

READY. SET. REVIEW.
Online and on the Go!

Davis Mobile Apps

✓ iPhone ✓ iPod Touch ✓ iPad ✓ Android

1,500+ questions for study on the go, including alternate-format items.

132 need-to-know 'high alert' drugs on flash cards with trade and generic names, classifications, and audio pronunciations.

389 of the most prescribed generic drugs on flash cards detailing drug action, indication, pre-administration vital signs, laboratory data assessment, drug levels, and patient teaching.

Online Testing

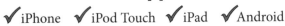

DAVISReview
OHMAN'S NCLEX-RN® PREP

Comprehensive online testing program simulating the actual exam with test-taking tips, rationales for every response, and performance analysis.

Visit www.FADavis.com for more information.
Keyword: **Davis Mobile** / Keyword: **Davis Review**

www.FADavis.com

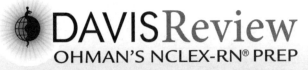

abobotulinumtoxinA
(ab-oh-**bot**-yoo-**lye**-num **tox**-in ay)
Dysport

Classification
Thera: antispasticity agents, cosmetic agents
Pharm: neurotoxins

Pregnancy Category C

Indications
Treatment of cervical dystonia in adults in order to ↓ severity of abnormal head position and neck pain. Temporary improvement of moderate to severe glabellar (frown) lines in adult patients <65 yr.

Action
Inhibits release of acetylcholine from peripheral cholinergic nerve endings, resulting chemical denervation of treated muscle. **Therapeutic Effects:** Localized reduction of muscle activity, with ↓ spasticity in cervical dystonia. ↓ appearance of glabellar lines.

Pharmacokinetics
Absorption: Minimal but may be significant in selected populations.
Distribution: Unknown.
Metabolism and Excretion: Unknown.
Half-life: Unknown.

TIME/ACTION PROFILE (improvement in spasticity/appearance of lines)

ROUTE	ONSET	PEAK	DURATION
IM	within 4 wk	unknown	up to 4 mo

Contraindications/Precautions
Contraindicated in: Hypersensitivity to botulinum toxin products or additives; Allergy to cow's-milk protein; Infection at injection site.
Use Cautiously in: Previous surgical facial alterations, marked facial asymmetry, known weakness/atrophy of muscle in question, inflammation or skin abnormality at injection site, ptosis; Peripheral motor neuropathic disorders (may exacerbate clinical effects and ↑ the risk of severe dysphagia and respiratory compromise); Hyperhydrosis (safe use not established); Geri: Use cautiously; consider concurrent diseases and drug therapy; OB: Use during pregnancy only if potential benefit justifies potential risk to the fetus; Pedi: Safe and effective use in children <18 yr has not been established.

Adverse Reactions/Side Effects
Cervical dsytonia
CNS: fatigue, headache. **EENT:** dysphonia, eye disorder. **GI:** dry mouth, dysphagia. **Local:** injection site pain. **MS:** muscular weaknesson, neck pain. **Misc:** SPREAD OF TOXIN EFFECT.

Glabellar lines
CNS: headache. **EENT:** nasopharyngitis, eyelid edema, eyelid ptosis, sinusitus. **Resp:** nasopharyngitis, dyspnea. **GI:** nausea, dysphagia. **Local:** injection site pain/reaction. **Misc:** SPREAD OF TOXIN EFFECT.

Interactions
Drug-Drug: Concurrent use of **aminoglycosides** or other **agents interfering with neuromuscular transmission** including **curare-like agents** or **muscle relaxants** may ↑ effect. Concurrent use of **anticholinergics** ↑ systemic anticholinergic effects.

Route/Dosage
Cervical dystonia
IM (Adults): 500 Units as a divided dose among affected muscles; may be repeated every 12–16 wk, based on return of symptoms (range 250 and 1000 Units). Increments may be made in 250 Unit steps according to response.

Glabellar lines
IM (Adults <65 yr): 50 Units, divided in five equal aliquots of 10 Units; may be repeated every 3 mo.

Availability
Freeze dried powder for reconstitution: 500 Unit vial, 300 Unit vial.

♣ = Canadian drug name. ☒ = Genetic implication.
*CAPITALS indicates life-threatening; <u>underlines</u> indicate most frequent.

NURSING IMPLICATIONS

Assessment

- Assess heart rate in patients with history of heart disease. May cause a slight (3 beats per minute) reduction in heart rate 30 min following injection.
- **Cervical Dystonia:** Assess amount of spasticity prior to and following therapy.
- **Glabellar Lines:** Assess level of glabellar lines prior to and following therapy.
- **Lab Test Considerations:** May cause slight ↑ of blood glucose.

Potential Nursing Diagnoses

Impaired physical mobility (Indications)
Disturbed body image (Indications)

Implementation

- The potency Units of abobotulinumtoxinA are not interchangeable with other botulinum toxin products.

Cervical Dystonia

- **IM:** Reconstitute each single-use 500 mg vial with 1 mL or 300 mg vial with 0.6 mL of 0.9% NaCl without preservatives. **Concentration:** 500 mg/mL or 250 mg/mL, respectively Swirl gently to dissolve. Solution should be clear and colorless; do not administer solutions that are discolored or contain particulate matter. Refrigerate solution and protect from light; do not freeze. Administer into affected muscles within 4 hrs using a 23 or 25 gauge needle. Discard remaining solution.

Glabellar Lines

- **IM:** Reconstitute each 300 mg vial with 2.5 mL or 1.5 mL of 0.9% NaCl without preservatives. **Concentration:** 10 Units/0.8 mL or 10 Units/0.5 mL, respectively Using a 21 gauge needle, insert at a 45° angle into abobotulinumtoxinA vial and allow the vacuum to pull 0.9% NaCl into vial. Discard vial if vacuum has been lost. Gently rotate until white substance is fully dissolved; do not shake. Solution should be clear and colorless; do not administer solutions that are discolored or contain particulate matter. Solution is stable for 4 hrs if refrigerated and protected from light;

do not freeze. Draw up single dose and expel any air bubbles in syringe barrel. Exchange needle for a 30 gauge needle for administration. Administer 5 equally divided aliquots of 10 Units each into 5 sites (2 in each corrugator muscle, 1 in procerus muscle).

Patient/Family Teaching

- Inform patient of purpose of abotulinumtoxinA Advise patient to read *Patient Medication Guide* prior to treatment.
- Inform patient that effects of abotulinumtoxinA may spread beyond the site of local injection. Advise patient to notify health care professional immediately if problems swallowing, speaking, or breathing occur or if signs and symptoms of spread (asthenia, generalized muscle weakness, diplopia, blurred vision, ptosis, dysphagia, dysarthria, urinary incontinence, breathing difficulties) occur. May occur hrs to wks after injection.
- May cause loss of strength, muscle weakness, blurred vision, or drooping eyelids. Caution patient to avoid driving and other activities requiring alertness until response to medication is known.
- Instruct patient to notify health care professional of all Rx or OTC medications, vitamins, or herbal products being taken and consult health care professional before taking any new medications.
- Advise female patients to notify health care professional if pregnancy is planned or suspected or if breastfeeding.

Evaluation/Desired Outcomes

- Localized reduction of muscle activity, with ↓ spasticity in cervical dystonia.
- ↓ appearance of glabellar lines.

**acetaminophen
(intravenous)**
(a-seet-a-**min**-oh-fen)
Ofirmev

Indications

Treatment of mild to moderate pain. With opioid analgesics for the treatment of moderate to severe pain. Reduction of fever.

Action

Inhibits the synthesis of prostaglandins that may serve as mediators of pain and fever, primarily in the CNS. Has no significant anti-inflammatory properties or GI toxicity. **Therapeutic Effects:** Analgesia. Antipyresis.

Pharmacokinetics

Absorption: Intravenous administration results in complete bioavailability.
Distribution: Widely distributed. Crosses the placenta; enters breast milk in low concentrations.
Metabolism and Excretion: 85–95% metabolized by the liver (CYP2E1 enzyme system). Metabolites may be toxic in overdose situation. Metabolites excreted by the kidneys.
Half-life: *Adults*— 2.4 hr, *adolescents*— 2.9 hr, *children*— 3.0 hr, *infants*— 4.2 hr, *neonates*— 2.7 hr.

TIME/ACTION PROFILE (effect on fever)

ROUTE	ONSET	PEAK	DURATION
IV	within 30 min	30 min	4–6 hr

Contraindications/Precautions

Contraindicated in: Hypersensitivity; Severe hepatic impairment/active liver disease.
Use Cautiously in: Hepatic impairment/active liver disease (↓ daily dose recommended), alcoholism, chronic malnutrition, severe hypovolemia or severe renal impairment (CCr <30 mL/min, ↑ dosing interval and ↓ daily dose may be

necessary); OB: Use in pregnancy only if clearly needed; Lactation: Use cautiously; Pedi: Safe and effective use in children <2 yr not established.

Adverse Reactions/Side Effects

CNS: agitation (↑ in children), anxiety, headache, fatigue, insomnia. **Resp:** atelectasis (↑ in children), dyspnea. **CV:** hypertension, hypotension. **GI:** HEPATOTOXICITY (↑ DOSES), constipation (↑ in children), ↑ liver enzymes, nausea, vomiting. **Derm:** pruritus (↑ in children). **F and E:** hypokalemia. **MS:** muscle spasms, trismus.

Interactions

Drug-Drug: Chronic doses >4000 mg/day may ↑ risk of bleeding from **warfarin**. Drugs that induce/regulate the **CYP2E1 enzyme system** may ↑ production of a toxic metabolite and risk of adverse reactions.

Route/Dosage

IV (Adults and adolescents ≥50 kg): 1000 mg every six hr or 650 mg every four hr (not to exceed 4000 mg/day or less than four hour dosing interval).
IV (Adults and adolescents <50 kg): 15 mg/kg every six hr or 12.5 mg/kg every four hr (not to exceed 75 mg/kg/day or less than 4 hour dosing interval).
IV (Children 2–12 yr): 15 mg/kg every six hr or 12.5 mg/kg every every four hr (not to exceed 75 mg/kg/day or less than 4 hour dosing interval).

Availability

Solution for intravenous infusion: 1000 mg/100 mL in 100-mL vials.

NURSING IMPLICATIONS

Assessment

● Assess overall health status and alcohol usage before administering acetaminophen. Patients who are malnourished or chronically abuse alcohol are at higher risk of developing hepatotoxicity with chronic use of usual doses of acetaminophen.

- **Pain:** Assess type, location, and intensity prior to and 30 min following administration.
- **Fever:** Assess fever; note presence of associated signs (diaphoresis, tachycardia, and malaise).
- *Lab Test Considerations:* ↑ serum bilirubin, LDH, AST, ALT, and prothrombin time may indicate hepatotoxicity.
- *Toxicity and Overdose:* If overdose occurs, acetylcysteine (Acetadote) is the antidote.

Potential Nursing Diagnoses
Acute pain (Indications)
Risk for imbalanced body temperature (Indications)

Implementation

IV Administration

- **Intermittent Infusion:** *For 1000 mg dose,* insert vented IV set through septum of 100 mL vial; may be administered without further dilution. *For doses <1000 mg,* withdraw appropriate dose from vial place in a separate empty, sterile container for IV infusion. Place small volume pediatric doses up to 60 mL in a syringe and administer via syringe pump. Solution is clear and colorless; do not administer solutions that are discolored of contain particulate matter. Administer within 6 hrs of breaking vial seal. *Rate:* Infuse over 15 min. Monitor end of infusion in order to prevent air embolism, especially if acetaminophen is primary infusion.
- **Y-Site Incompatibility:** chlorpromazine, diazepam.
- **Additive Incompatibility:** Do not mix with other medications.

Patient/Family Teaching
- Explain purpose of acetaminophen to patient.
- Advise patient to consult health care professional if discomfort or fever is not relieved.

Evaluation/Desired Outcomes
- Relief of mild pain.
- Reduction of fever.

alglucosidase
(al-gloo-ko-**side**-ase)
Lumizyme, Myozyme

Classification
Thera: replacement enzyme

Pregnancy Category B

Indications
Myozyme: Replacement enzyme in infantile-onset Pompe disease (alpha glucosidase (GAA) deficiency). **Lumizyme**: Replacement enzyme in late-onset (noninfantile) Pompe disease in patients without evidence of cardiac hypertrophy.

Action
Replaces alpha-glucosidase. Without this enzyme, glycogen accumulates in tissues including cardiac and skeletal muscles and hepatic tissues, leading to the development of cardiomyopathy, progressive muscle weakness, and impairment of respiratory function. **Therapeutic Effects:** Improved survival with delayed need for ventilatory support. Improved lung function and exercise capacity.

Pharmacokinetics
Absorption: IV administration results in complete bioavailability.
Distribution: Unknown.
Metabolism and Excretion: Unknown.
Half-life: 2.3–2.5 hr.

TIME/ACTION PROFILE

ROUTE	ONSET	PEAK	DURATION
IV	unknown	end of infusion	2 wks

Contraindications/Precautions
Contraindicated in: None known.
Use Cautiously in: Acute underlying illness (↑ risk of infusion reactions); OB: Use only if clearly needed; Lactation: Lactation; Pedi: Safety not established in children <1 mo or >3.5 yr (Myozyme) or <8 yr (Lumizyme).

Adverse Reactions/Side Effects

CV: <u>bradycardia</u>, <u>tachycardia</u>. **Resp:** RESPIRATORY DISTRESS FAILURE, <u>cough</u>, ↓ <u>oxygen saturation</u>, tachypnea. **EENT:** blurred vision, vertigo. **GI:** <u>constipation</u>, <u>diarrhea</u>, <u>reflux</u>, <u>vomiting</u>. **Derm:** NECROTIZING SKIN LESIONS, <u>flushing</u>, <u>rash</u>, dermatitis, urticaria. **Hemat:** <u>anemia</u>, lymphadenopathy. **F and E:** edema. **Misc:** allergic reactions including ANAPHYLAXIS, INFUSION REACTIONS, <u>fever</u>.

Interactions

Drug-Drug: None noted.

Route/Dosage

IV (Children 1 mo–3.5 yr): *Myozyme*— 20 mg/kg every 2 wks.
IV (Adults and Children ≥8 yr): *Lumizyme*— 20 mg/kg every 2 wks.

Availability

Lyophilized powder for IV administration (requires reconstitution): 50 mg/vial.

NURSING IMPLICATIONS

Assessment

- Observe for signs and symptoms of anaphylaxis (rash, pruritus, laryngeal edema, wheezing). Keep epinephrine, an antihistamine, corticosteroids, and resuscitation equipment close by in case of anaphylactic reaction.
- Monitor for infusion-related reactions (headache, fever, tachycardia, cough, cyanosis, rash, erythema, urticaria, hypotension. Most reactions are managed with antihistamines and/or corticosteroids prior to or during infusions, slowing rate of infusion, and/or early discontinuation if reaction is serious. Infusion reactions may occur any time during or up to 2 hr after infusion and are more likely with higher infusion rates.
- Monitor cardiorespiratory status continuously during therapy. May cause acute cardiorespiratory failure requiring intubation and inotropic support.

- ***Lab Test Considerations:*** Monitor liver enzymes prior to and periodically during therapy.

Potential Nursing Diagnoses

Ineffective tissue perfusion (Indications)

Implementation

- *Lumizyme* is available only through a restricted distribution program called the LUMIZYME ACE Program due to the potential risk of rapid disease progression in Pompe disease patients less than 8 yrs of age. Only prescribers and healthcare facilities enrolled in the program may prescribe, dispense or administer *Lumizyme*. *Lumizyme* may be administered only to patients who are enrolled in and meet all the conditions of the *Lumizyme ACE* Program. To enroll in the *Lumizyme ACE* Program call 1-800-745-4447.

IV Administration

- **Intermittent Infusion:** Determine number of vials required for the dose ordered. If number of vials includes a fraction, round up to next whole number. Allow vials to reach room temperature before reconstitution, approximately 30 min. Reconstitute by slowly injecting 10.3 mL of Sterile Water for Injection to inside wall of each vial. Avoid forceful impact of water on powder to avoid foaming. Tilt and roll each vial gently. Do not invert, swirl, or shake. Protect solution from light. Each vial contains 5 mg/mL with a total extractable dose of 50 mg/10 mL. Solution is clear and may occasionally contain white strands or translucent fibers; do not administer solutions that are discolored or contain particulate matter. Vials are for single use; discard remaining medication. ***Diluent:*** Dilute each vial in 100 mL of 0.9% NaCl immediately after reconstitution. ***Concentration:*** 0.5–4 mg/mL Slowly withdraw reconstituted solution from each vial. Remove airspace from infusion bag to minimize particle formation due to sensitivity of medication to air. Add reconstituted solution slowly and directly into 0.9% NaCl solution, not into airspace in bag. Gently invert or massage to mix; do not shake. Use a 0.2 micrometer low-protein binding in-line filter for administration. Administer immediately. Solution may be stored in refrigerator for up to 24 hr. *Rate:* Administer over 4 hr. Using an infusion pump, administer initially at a rate of 1 mg/kg/hr. ↑ rate to 2 mg/kg/hr every 30 min, after tolerance to medication is established, until a maximum rate of 7 mg/kg/hr is reached. Monitor vital signs with each dose ↑. If stable, administer at 7 mg/kg/hr until infusion is completed. Slow or temporarily stop infusion if infusion reactions occur.

Patient/Family Teaching
● Inform patient that a registry for patients with Pompe disease was established to evaluate long term treatments. Women of childbearing potential are also encouraged to register. For information, visit www.pomperegistry.com or call 1-800-745-4447.

Evaluation/Desired Outcomes
● Improved survival with delayed need for ventilatory support in patients with Pompe disease.
● Improved lung function and exercise capacity.

azilsartan
(a-zill-**sar**-tan)
Edarbi

Classification
Thera: antihypertensives
Pharm: angiotensin II receptor antagonists

Pregnancy Category C (first trimester), D (second and third trimesters)

Indications
Treatment of hypertension, alone or with other agents.

Action
Blocks vasoconstrictor and aldosterone-producing effects of angiotensin II at receptor sites, including vascular smooth muscle and the adrenal glands. **Therapeutic Effects:** Lowering of blood pressure.

Pharmacokinetics
Absorption: Azilsartan medoxomil, a prodrug, in hydrolized in the GI tract to azilsartan, the active component. 60% is absorbed from the GI tract.
Distribution: Approximately 16 L.
Protein Binding: ≥99%.
Metabolism and Excretion: 50% metabolized by the liver, primarily by the CYP2C9 enzyme system. 55% eliminated in feces, 42% in urine (15% an unchanged azlisartan).
Half-life: 11 hr.

TIME/ACTION PROFILE (effect on blood pressure)

ROUTE	ONSET	PEAK	DURATION
PO	within 2 hr	18 hr	24 hr

Contraindications/Precautions
Contraindicated in: OB: Can cause injury or death of fetus; Lactation: Discontinue drug or provide formula.
Use Cautiously in: ⚖ Black patients (may not be effective); CHF (may result in potentially life-threatening renal failure); Renal impairment; may worsen renal function; Volume or salt depletion, including use of high-dose or potent diuretics may ↑ risk of serious hypotension; correct prior to use; Woman of childbearing potential; Geri: May have greater sensitivity, especially to adverse renal effects; Pedi: Safe and effective use in children has not been established.

Adverse Reactions/Side Effects
CNS: dizziness, fatigue, weakness. **Resp:** cough. **CV:** hypotension. **GI:** diarrhea, nausea. **MS:** muscle spasm.

Interactions
Drug-Drug: Concurrent use of **NSAIDs** may ↑ risk of/worsen renal impairment. Antihypertensive effect may be blunted by **NSAIDs**. ↑ antihypertensive effect with other **antihypertensives** or **diuretics**.

Route/Dosage

PO (Adults): 80 mg once daily, initial dose may be lowered to 40 mg once daily if high doses of diuretics are used concurrently.

Availability

Tablets: 40 mg, 80 mg.

NURSING IMPLICATIONS

Assessment

- Assess blood pressure (sitting, lying, standing) and pulse periodically during therapy.
- Monitor frequency of prescription refills to determine adherence to therapy.
- *Lab Test Considerations:* Monitor renal function. May cause small, reversible ↑ serum creatinine. May cause worsening renal function in patients with renal impairment. May rarely cause slight ↓ in RBC, hemoglobin and hematocrit.
- May cause low and high markedly abnormal platelet and WBC.

Potential Nursing Diagnoses

Risk for injury (Adverse Reactions)
Noncompliance (Patient/Family Teaching)

Implementation

- Correct volume and salt depletion, if possible, before initiation of therapy, or start treatment at 40 mg.
- **PO:** Administer once daily without regard to food.

Patient/Family Teaching

- Emphasize the importance of continuing to take as directed, even if feeling well. Take missed doses as soon as remembered if not almost before next dose; do not double doses. Medication controls but does not cure hypertension. Instruct patient to take medication at the same time each day. Warn patient not to discontinue therapy unless directed by health care professional.
- Encourage patient to comply with additional interventions for hypertension (weight reduction, low-sodium diet, smoking cessation, moderation of alcohol consumption, regular exercise, and stress management). Medication controls but does not cure hypertension.
- Instruct patient and family on proper technique for monitoring blood pressure. Advise them to check blood pressure at least weekly and to report significant changes.
- Caution patient to avoid sudden position changes to ↓ orthostatic hypotension. Use of alcohol, standing for long periods, exercising, and hot weather may ↑ orthostatic hypotension.
- May cause dizziness. Caution patient to avoid driving and other activities requiring alertness until response to medication is known.
- Instruct patient to notify health care professional of all Rx or OTC medications, vitamins, or herbal products being taken and to avoid concurrent use of Rx, OTC, and herbal products, especially NSAIDs and cough, cold, or allergy medications, without consulting health care professional.
- Instruct patient to notify health care professional of medication regimen before treatment or surgery.
- Emphasize the importance of follow-up exams to evaluate effectiveness of medication.
- Advise women of childbearing age to use contraception and notify health care professional if pregnancy is planned or suspected, or if breastfeeding. Azilsartan should be discontinued as soon as possible when pregnancy is detected.

Evaluation/Desired Outcomes

- ↓ in blood pressure without excessive side effects.

belimumab
(be-**li**-moo-mab)
Benlysta

Classification
Thera: immunosuppressants
Pharm: monoclonal antibodies

Pregnancy Category C

Indications
Treatment of active autoantibody-positive systemic lupus erythematosus (SLE) in patients currently receiving standard therapy.

Action
A monoclonal antibody produced by recombinant DNA technique that specifically binds to B lymphocyte stimulator protein (BLyS), thereby inactivating it. **Therapeutic Effects:** ↓ survival of B cells, including auroreactive ones and ↓ differentiation into immunoglobulin-producing plasma cells. Result is ↓ disease activity with lessened damage/improvement in mucocutaneous, musculoskeletal and immunologic manifestations of SLE.

Pharmacokinetics
Absorption: IV administration results in complete bioavailability.
Distribution: Unknown.
Metabolism and Excretion: Unknown.
Half-life: 19.4 days.

TIME/ACTION PROFILE (reduction in activated B cells)

ROUTE	ONSET	PEAK	DURATION
IV	8 wk	unknown	52 wk†

†With continuous treatment.

Contraindications/Precautions
Contraindicated in: Hypersensitivity; Concurrent use of other biologicals or cyclophosphamide; Concurrent use of live vaccines; Lactation: Breast-feeding not recommended.
Use Cautiously in: Infections (consider temporary withdrawal for acute infections, treat aggressively); Previous history of depression or suicidal ideation (may worsen); Geri: may be more sensitive to drug effects, consider age-related changes in renal, hepatic and cardiac function, concurrent drug therapy and chronic disease states; OB: Use during pregnancy only if potential maternal benefit outweighs potential fetal risk; women with childbearing potential should use adequate contraception during and for four months following treatment.

Adverse Reactions/Side Effects
CNS: depression, insomnia, migraine. **GI:** nausea, diarrhea. **GU:** cystitis. **Hemat:** leukopenia. **MS:** extremity pain. **Misc:** allergic reactions including ANAPHYLAXIS, INFECTION, infusion reactions, fever.

Interactions
Drug-Drug: ↑ risk of adverse reactions and ↓ immune response to **live vaccines**; should not be given concurrently.

Route/Dosage
PO (Adults): 10 mg/kg every two wks for three doses, then every four wks.

Availability
Lyophilized powder for IV administration (requires reconstitution and dilution: 120 mg/vial, 400 mg/vial.

NURSING IMPLICATIONS

Assessment
- Monitor patient for signs of anaphylaxis (hypotension, angioedema, urticaria, rash, pruritus, wheezing, dyspnea, facial edema) during and following injection. Medications (antihistamines, corticosteroids, epinephrine) and equipment should be readily available in the event of a severe reaction. Discontinue belimumab immediately if anaphylaxis or other severe allergic reaction occurs.
- Monitor for infusion reactions (headache, nausea, skin reactions, bradycardia, myalgia, headache, rash, urticaria, hypotension). There is insufficient evidence to determine whether premedication diminishes frequency or severity. Infusion rate may be slowed or interrupted if an infusion reaction occurs.
- Assess for signs of infection (fever, dyspnea, flu-like symptoms, frequent or painful urination, redness or swelling at the site of a wound), including tuberculosis, prior to injection. Belimumab is

contraindicated in patients with active infection. New infections should be monitored closely; most common are upper respiratory tract infections, bronchitis, and urinary tract infections. Signs and symptoms of inflammation may be lessened due to suppression from belimumab. Infections may be fatal, especially in patients taking immunosuppressive therapy. If patient develops a serious infection, consider discontinuing belimumab until infection is controlled.

- Assess mental status and mood changes. Inform health care professional if patient demonstrates significant ↑ in depressed mood, anxiety, nervousness, or insomnia.

Potential Nursing Diagnoses
Risk for infection (Adverse Reactions)

Implementation
- Consider premedication for prophylaxis against infusion reactions and hypersensitivity reactions.

IV Administration
- **Intermittent Infusion:** Remove belimumab from refrigerator and allow to stand 10–15 min to reach room temperature. Reconstitute 120 mg vial with 1.5 mL and 400 mg vial with 4.8 mL of Sterile Water for Injection by directing stream toward side if vial to minimize foaming. Swirl gently for 60 seconds. Allow vial to site at room temperature during reconstitution, swirling gently for 60 seconds every 5 min until powder is dissolved. Do not shake. Reconstitution usually takes 10–15 min, but may take up to 30 min. Protect from sunlight. Solution is opalescent and colorless to pale yellow and without particles. Small bubbles are expected and acceptable. *Concentration:* 80 mg/mL. *Diluent:* 0.9% NaCL. Remove volume of patient's dose from a 250 mL infusion bag and discard. Replace with required amount of reconstituted solution. Gently invert bag to mix. Do not administer solutions that are discolored

or contain particulate matter. Discard unused solution in vial. If not used immediately, refrigerate and protect from light. Solution is stable for 8 hrs. *Rate:* Infuse over 1 hr; may slow or interrupt rate if patient develops an infusion reaction.

- **Y-Site Incompatibility:** Do not administer with dextrose solutions or other solutions or medications.

Patient/Family Teaching
- Instruct patient to read *Medication Guide* prior to each treatment session.
- Caution patient to notify health care professional immediately if signs of infection (fever, sweating, chills, muscle aches, cough, shortness of breath, blood in phlegm, weight loss, warm, red or painful skin or sores, diarrhea or stomach pain, burning on urination, urinary frequency, feeling tired), severe rash, swollen face, or difficulty breathing occurs while taking.
- Advise patient to report signs and symptoms of anaphylaxis to health care professional immediately.
- Advise patient, family, and caregivers to look for depression and suicidality, especially during early therapy or dose changes. Notify health care professional immediately if thoughts about suicide or dying, attempts to commit suicide; new or worse depression or anxiety; agitation or restlessness; panic attacks; insomnia; new or worse irritability; aggressiveness; acting on dangerous impulses, mania, or other changes in mood or behavior or if symptoms of serotonin syndrome occur.
- Caution patient to avoid receiving live vaccines for 30 days before and during belimumab therapy.
- Advise women of childbearing potential to use adequate contraception and to avoid breastfeeding during and for at least 4 mos after final treatment.

Evaluation/Desired Outcomes
- Improvement in mucocutaneous, musculoskeletal, and immunologic disease activity in patients with SLE.

benzyl alcohol
(**ben**-zill **al**-ko-hol)
Ulesfia

Classification
Thera: pediculocides

Pregnancy Category B

Indications
Topical treatment of head lice in patients ≥6 mo.

Action
Kills head lice (pediculocidal); not ovocidal. **Therapeutic Effects:** Eradication of head lice.

Pharmacokinetics
Absorption: Minimal absorption follows recommended application.
Distribution: Unknown.
Metabolism and Excretion: Unknown.
Half-life: Unknown.

TIME/ACTION PROFILE

ROUTE	ONSET	PEAK	DURATION
Topical	rapid	unknown	unknown

Contraindications/Precautions
Contraindicated in: None noted; Pedi: Children <6 mo (safety not established; risk of gasping syndrome in neonates).
Use Cautiously in: OB: Lactation.

Adverse Reactions/Side Effects
EENT: ocular irritation. **Derm:** contact dermatitis, erythema, pruritus, pyoderma. **Local:** application site anesthesia, application site hypoesthesia, application site irritation, pain.

Interactions
Drug-Drug: None noted.

Route/Dosage
Topical (Adults and Children ≥6 mo): *Short hair 0–2 in long*—apply 4–6 oz (1/2–3/4 bottle) repeat in 7 days; *Short hair 2–4 in long*—apply 6–8 oz (3/4–1 bottle) repeat in 7 days; *Medium hair 4–8 in long*—apply 8–12 oz (1–1 1/2 bottles) repeat in 7 days; *Medium hair 8–16 in long*—apply 12–24 oz (1 1/2–3 bottles), repeat in 7 days; *Long hair 16–22 in long*—apply 24–32 oz (3–4 bottles), repeat in 7 days; *Long hair >22 in long*—apply 32–48 oz (4–6 bottles), repeat in 7 days.

Availability
5% lotion: in 8-oz bottles.

NURSING IMPLICATIONS

Assessment
● Assess for signs of head lice prior to and following treatment.

Potential Nursing Diagnoses
Risk for impaired skin integrity (Indications)
Deficient knowledge, related to medication regimen (Patient/Family Teaching)

Implementation
● **Topical:** Cover face and eyes with a towel and keep eyes tightly closed. Apply lotion to *dry* hair, using enough to completely saturate scalp and hair. Massage lotion into hair and scalp and behind ears. Leave on for 10 min and thoroughly rinse off with water. Repeat in 7 days Avoid contact with eyes. Wash hands after application. A fine-tooth comb may be used to remove dead nits from hair and scalp.

Patient/Family Teaching
● Instruct patient/parent to use benzyl alcohol as directed. If lotion comes in contact with eyes, flush them immediately with water. Notify health care professional if irritation persists. Emphasize the importance of second treatment 1 wk after initial application. Instruct patient/parent to read Patient Information before using benzyl alcohol and with each Rx refill; new information may be available.
● Advise patient/parent to wash in hot water or dry clean all recently worn clothing, hats, used bedding, and towels. Wash personal care items such as combs, brushes, and hair clips in hot water.
● Advise female patients or parents to notify health care professional if pregnancy is planned or suspected or if breast feeding.

Evaluation/Desired Outcomes
• Eradication of head lice.

buprenorphine/ naloxone
(boo-pre-**nor**-feen/na-**lox**-one)
Suboxone

Classification
Thera: agents for opioid addiction
Pharm: opioid agonists/antagonists, opioid antagonists

Schedule III

Pregnancy Category C

Indications
Maintenance treatment of opioid dependence as part of a comprehensive program including counseling and psychological support.

Action
Buprenorphine—Binds to opiate receptors in the CNS. *Sublingual naloxone*—has no pharmacological effect; it is present in the formulation to discourage injection of the product by opioid-dependent patients. **Therapeutic Effects:** Suppression of withdrawal symptoms during detoxification and maintenance from opioids.

Pharmacokinetics
Absorption: *Buprenorphine*—Well absorbed following SL administration; *naloxone*—Negligable absorption follows SL administration.
Distribution: *Buprenorphine*—Crosses the placenta; enters breast milk. CNS concentration is 15–25% of plasma.
Protein Binding: *Buprenorphine*—Protein Binding: 96%.
Metabolism and Excretion: *Buprenorphine*—Mostly metabolized by the liver mostly via the CYP3A4 enzyme system; one metabolite is active; 70% excreted in feces; 27% excreted in urine.
Half-life: *Buprenorphine*—33 hr; *Naloxone*—60–90 min (up to 3 hr in neonates).

TIME/ACTION PROFILE

ROUTE	ONSET	PEAK†	DURATION
SL buprenorphine	unknown	1.5–1.7 hr	24 hr

† Blood level.

Contraindications/Precautions
Contraindicated in: Hypersensitivity to buprenorphine or naloxone; Lactation: Buprenorphine enters breast milk; avoid breast-feeding.
Use Cautiously in: Compromised respiratory function including COPD, cor pulmonale, diminished respiratory reserve, hypoxia, hypercapnia or respiratory depression of other causes; Geri: elderly or debilitated patients may be more sensitive to drug effects; OB: Buprenorphine crosses the placenta, use during pregnancy only if potential benefit justifies potential risk; Pedi: Safe use in children <16 yr not established.

Adverse Reactions/Side Effects
CNS: <u>headache</u>, <u>insomnia</u>. **CV:** orthostatic hypotension. **Resp:** RESPIRATORY DEPRESSION. **GI:** <u>constipation</u>, glossodynia, nausea, <u>oral hypoesthesia, oral mucosal erythema</u>, vomiting, hepatitis. **Derm:** <u>hyperhydrosis</u>. **F and E:** peripheral edema. **Misc:** allergic reactions including ANAPHYLAXIS, physical dependence, psychological dependence, tolerance, withdrawal phenomenon.

Interactions
Drug-Drug: Use with extreme caution in patients receiving **MAO inhibitors** (↑ CNS and respiratory depression and hypotension— ↓ buprenorphine dose by 50%; may need to ↓ **MAO inhibitor** dose. Inhibitors of the CYP3A4 enzyme system including **itraconazole, ketoconazole, erythromycin, ritonavir, indinavir, saquinavir, atazanavir**, or

fosamprenavir may ↑ blood levels and effects; may need to ↓ buprenorphine dose. Blood levels/effects may be ↓ and withdrawal may be initiated by **inducers of the CYP3A4 enzyme system** including **carbamazepine**, **phenobarbital**, **phenytoin** or **rifampicin**; dose alterations may be necessary. ↑ risk of CNS depression with other **CNS depressants** including **alcohol**, **antihistamines**, **benzodiazepines**, **phenothiazines**, **sedative/hypnotics**, and some **antidepressants**; dose adjustments may necessary.

Drug-Natural Products: Concomitant use of **kava-kava**, **valerian**, **chamomile**, or **hops** can ↑ CNS depression.

Route/Dosage

SL (Adults): Progressively ↑ /adjusted in increments of buprenorphine 2 mg/naloxone 0.5 mg or buprenorphine 4 mg/naloxone 1 mg. Titrate to keep patient engaged in treatment while suppressing opioid withdrawal; usual target dose is buprenorphine 16 mg/naloxone 4 mg once daily.

Availability

Sublingual film (lime-flavored): buprenorphine 2 mg/naloxone 0.5 mg per film, buprenorphine 8 mg/naloxone 2 mg per film.

NURSING IMPLICATIONS

Assessment

- During initial therapy, assess patient at least weekly during first month and frequently thereafter for compliance, effectiveness of treatment plan, and overall patient progress. Once a stable dose is achieved, monthly assessment may be used. Determine absence of medication toxicity, medical, or behavioral adverse effect; responsible handling of medications by patient; compliance with treatment plan including recovery-oriented activities and psychotherapy or other modalities; abstinence from illicit drug use.
- *Lab Test Considerations:* Monitor liver function test prior to beginning therapy and periodically during treatment.

Potential Nursing Diagnoses

Ineffective coping (Indications)

Implementation

- Buprenorphine/naloxone sublingual film is not appropriate as an analgesic.
- Can only be prescribed by clinicians who meet qualifying requirements, and who have notified the Secretary of Health and Human Services of their intent to prescribe this product for the treatment of opioid dependence and have been assigned a unique identification number that must be included on every prescription.
- Induction of therapy begins with patient being in a moderate state of opioid withdrawal and receiving buprenorphine for 2–3 days. Once the induction phase is completed, maintenance begins with buprenorphine/naloxone titration.
- Patients receiving buprenorphine/naloxone sublingual tablets may be switched to sublingual film of same dose. Dose adjustments may be required.
- **SL:** Place film under tongue. If additional film is required for dose, place on opposite side of tongue from first film, minimizing overlap. Keep film under tongue until dissolved (5–7 min); do not chew, swallow, or move after placement.

Patient/Family Teaching

- Instruct patient to take medication as directed. Do not take more often than prescribed and consult health care professional before stopping; dose should be ↓ gradually to prevent withdrawal syndrome. Instruct patient to read *Medication Guide* before starting therapy and with each Rx refill. Advise patient to keep medication in a safe place, out of reach of children and protected from being stolen and do not share with others, even if they have the same symptoms. Explain that buprenorphine/naloxone sublingual film may be fatal to children and individuals not tolerant to opioids. Advise patient that selling or giving medication away is against the law.

- To dispose of unused films, remove from foil pouch and drop each film into toilet and flush.
- Caution patient of the danger of taking non-prescribed benzodiazepines or other CNS depressants, including alcohol, during therapy.
- May cause dizziness. Caution patient to avoid driving and other activities requiring alertness until response to medication is known.
- Advise patient to make position changes slowly to prevent orthostatic hypotension.
- Advise female patients to notify health care professional if pregnancy is planned or suspected, or if breastfeeding.
- Instruct patient to inform family that, in the event of an emergency, treating health care professionals should be informed that patient is physically dependent on an opioid and being treated with buprenorphine/naloxone sublingual film.

Evaluation/Desired Outcomes

- Maintenance treatment of opioid dependency.

cabazitaxel
(ka-ba-zi-**tax**-el)
Jevtana

Classification
Thera: antineoplastics
Pharm: taxoidsantimicrotubulars

Pregnancy Category D

Indications
Hormone-refractory metastatic prostate cancer previously treated with a regimen including docetaxel (used in combination with prednisone).

Action
Binds to intracellular tubulin and promotes its assembly into microtubules while inhibiting disassembly. Result is inhibition of mitotis and interphase. **Therapeutic Effects:** Death of rapidly replicating cells, particularly malignant ones, with ↓ spread of metastatic prostate cancer.

Pharmacokinetics
Absorption: IV administration results in complete bioavailability.
Distribution: Equally distributed between blood and plasma.
Metabolism and Excretion: Extensively (>95%) metabolized by the liver, 80–90% by CYP3A4/5 enzyme system. Metabolites are excreted in urine and feces. Minimal renal excretion.
Half-life: *Terminal elimination*—95 hr.

TIME/ACTION PROFILE (blood levels)

ROUTE	ONSET	PEAK	DURATION
IV	rapid	end of infusion	unknown

Contraindications/Precautions
Contraindicated in: Severe hypersensitivity to cabazitaxel or polysorbate 80; Neutrophils ≤1,500/mm³; Hepatic impairment (total bilirubin ≥upper limits of normal, or AST and/or ALT ≥1.5 × upper limits of normal); Concurrent use of strong CYP3A4 inhibitors, inducers and St. John's wort; OB: Avoid use during pregnancy (may cause fetal harm); Lactation: Breastfeeding should be avoided.
Use Cautiously in: Concurrent use of moderate CYP3A4 inhibitors; OB: Patients with child-bearing potential (pregnancy should be avoided); Patients with severe renal impairment (CCr <30 mL/min) or end-stage renal disease; Geri: Patients >65 yr ↑ risk of adverse reactions; Pedi: Safe and effective use in children has not been established.

Adverse Reactions/Side Effects
CNS: weakness, fatigue. **Resp:** dyspnea. **CV:** arrhythmias, hypotension. **GI:** DIARRHEA, abdominal pain, abnormal taste, anorexia, constipation, nausea, vomiting, dyspepsia. **GU:** RENAL FAILURE, hematuria. **Derm:** alopecia. **F and E:** electrolyte imbalance. **Hemat:** NEUTROPENIA, THROMBO-

CYTOPENIA, anemia, leukopenia. **MS:** arthralgia, back pain, muscle spasms.
Neuro: peripheral neuropathy. **Misc:** allergic reactions including ANAPHYLAXIS, fever.

Interactions

Drug-Drug: Concomitant administration of **strong CYP3A inhibitors** including **ketoconazole**, **itraconazole**, **clarithromycin**, **atazanavir**, **indinavir**, **nefazodone**, **nelfinavir**, **ritonavir**, **saquinavir**, **telithromycin** and **voriconazole** ↑ levels and risk of toxicity and should be avoided. Concomitant administration of **strong CYP3A inducers** including **phenytoin**, **carbamazepine**, **rifampin**, **rifabutin**, **rifapentin**, and **phenobarbital** may ↓ levels and effectiveness and should be avoided.

Drug-Natural Products: St. John's **wort** may ↓ levels and effectiveness and should be avoided.

Route/Dosage

PO (Adults): 25 mg/m² every three wks as a one-hour infusion (with prednisone 10 mg PO daily).

Availability

Viscous solution for injection (requires two dilutions prior to IV administration): 60 mg/1.5 mL (contains polysorbate 80) comes with diluent (5.7 mL of 13% [w/w] ethanol in water for injection).

NURSING IMPLICATIONS

Assessment

- Assess for hypersensitivity reactions (generalized rash/erythema, hypotension, bronchospasm, swelling of face). May occur within minutes following initiation of infusion. If severe reactions occur, discontinue infusion immediately and provide supportive therapy.
- Assess for nausea, vomiting, and severe diarrhea; may result in death due to electrolyte imbalance. Premedication is recommended. Treat with rehydration, anti-diarrheal, or antiemetic therapy as needed. If Grade ≥3 diarrhea or persisting diarrhea occurs despite appropriate medication, fluid and electrolyte

replacement, delay treatment until improvement or resolution, then reduce dose to 20 mg/mL.

- **Lab Test Considerations:** Monitor CBC weekly during cycle 1 and before each treatment cycle thereafter. Do not administer if neutrophils ≤1500/mm³. If prolonged grade 3 neutropenia (>1 wk) despite appropriate medication including filgrastim, delay treatment until neutrophil count is >1500 mm³, then reduce dose to 20 mg/m². Use filgrastim for secondary prophylaxis.
- If febrile neutropenia occurs, delay therapy until improvement or resolution and neutrophil count is >1500/mm³, then reduce dose to 20 mg/m². Use filgrastim for secondary prophylaxis.
- Discontinue cabazitaxel if prolonged Grade 3 neutropenia, febrile neutropenia or Grade 3 diarrhea occur at the 20 mg/m² dose.
- May cause hematuria.
- May cause Grade 3–4 ↑ AST, ↑ ALT, and ↑ bilirubin.

Potential Nursing Diagnoses

Risk for infection (Adverse Reactions)

Implementation

- **High Alert:** Fatalities have occurred with chemotherapeutic agents. Before administering, clarify all ambiguous orders; double check single, daily, and course-of-therapy dose limits; have second practitioner independently double check original order and dose calculations.
- Prepare solution in a biologic cabinet. Wear gloves, gown, and mask while handling medication. Discard equipment in specially designated containers. If solution comes in contact with skin or mucosa, wash with soap and water immediately.
- Premedicate at least 30 min before each dose with antihistamine (diphenhydramine 25 mg or equivalent), corticosteroid (dexamethasone 8 mg or equivalent) and H₂ antagonist (ranitidine 50 mg or equivalent). Antiemetic prophylaxis, PO or IV, is recommended.

IV Administration

- Two dilutions are required. Do not use PVC infusion containers or polyurethane infusion sets for preparation or infusion.
- **First Dilution: *Diluent:*** Mix vial with entire contents of supplied diluent-Direct needle to inside wall id vial and inject slowly to avoid foaming. Mix gently by repeated inversions for at least 45 seconds; do not shake. Let stand for a few minutes to allow foam to dissipate. *Concentration:* 10 mg/mL, **Second Dilution: *Diluent:***Withdraw recommended dose from cabazitaxel solution and dilute further into a setrile 250 mL PVC-free container of 0.9% NaCl or D5W. If dose >65 mg is required, use a larger volume of infusion vehicle so concentration does not exceed 0.26 mg/mL. Gently invert container to mix. *Concentration:* 0.10–0.26 mg/mL. Stable for 8 hrs (including 1 hr infusion) at room temperature or 24 hrs if refrigerated. May crystalize over time. Do not use if crystalized, discolored, or contains particulate matter; discard. *Rate:* Infuse over 1 hr at room temperature through a 0.22 micrometer nominal pore size filter.
- **Y-Site Incompatibility:** Do not mix with other medication.

Patient/Family Teaching

- Instruct patient to take oral prednisone as prescribed and to notify health care professional if a dose is missed or not taken in time.
- Advise patient to notify health care professional immediately if signs or symptoms of hypersensitivity reactions, fever; sore throat; signs of infection; lower back or side pain; difficult or painful urination; sores on the mouth or on the lips; bleeding gums; bruising; petechiae; blood in urine, stool, or emesis; unusual swelling occurs. Caution patient to avoid crowds and persons with known infections. Instruct patient to use soft toothbrush and electric razor and to avoid falls. Patient should also be cautioned not to drink alcoholic beverages or to take products containing aspirin or NSAIDs; may precipitate GI hemorrhage.
- Instruct patient to notify health care professional of all Rx or OTC medications, vitamins, or herbal products being taken and consult health care professional before taking any new medications.
- May cause dizziness. Caution patient to avoid driving or other activities requiring alertness until response to medication is known.
- Advise female patients of the need for contraception and to avoid breastfeeding during therapy.
- Instruct patient not to receive any vaccinations without advice of health care professional.
- Emphasize need for periodic lab tests to monitor for side effects. Advise patient to monitor temperature frequently.

Evaluation/Desired Outcomes

- ↓ in size and spread of metastatic prostate cancer.

---

carglumic acid
(car-**gloo**-mik **as**-id)
Carbaglu

Classification
Thera: hyperammonemia treatments (due to an enzyme deficiency)
Pharm: enzyme activators

Pregnancy Category C

Indications

Treatment (acute/maintenance) of hyperammonemia due to deficiency of hepatic enzyme N-acetylglutamate synthase (NAGS). During acute hyperammonemia, additional treatments should be used including alternate pathway medications, hemodialysis, and protein restriction.

Action

Serves as an analogue of N-acetyl gluta-mate (NAG), the natural activator of caba-moyl phosphate synthetase 1 (CPS 1) in the liver. CPS 1 helps to convert ammonia into urea. Carglumic acid replaces NAG in NAGS deficiency patients by activating CPS 1. **Therapeutic Effects:** ↓ ammonia levels.

Pharmacokinetics

Absorption: Some absorption follows oral administration; bioavailability unknown.

Distribution: Unknown.

Metabolism and Excretion: Some metabolism by intestinal bacteria; 9% excreted unchanged in urine, 60% excreted unchanged in feces. Metabolic end product (CO_2) eliminated via lungs.

Half-life: 5.6 hr.

TIME/ACTION PROFILE (↓ ammonia levels)

ROUTE	ONSET	PEAK	DURATION
PO	within 24 hr	3 days	unknown

Contraindications/Precautions

Contraindicated in: Lactation: Breast-feeding not recommended.

Use Cautiously in: OB: Due to risk of neurologic complications in NAGS patients, carglumic acid must be used throughout pregnancy.

Adverse Reactions/Side Effects

CNS: headache, drowsiness, weakness. **EENT:** nasopharyngitis. **GI:** abdominal pain, diarrhea, vomiting, abnormal taste. **Derm:** rash. **Hemat:** anemia. **Metab:** ↓ weight. **Misc:** infections, fever.

Interactions

Drug-Drug: None noted.

Route/Dosage

PO (Adults): 100–250 mg/kg/day initially, given in 2–4 divided doses immediately before meals/feedings, adjusted to maintain normal plasma ammonia levels based on age. Dose should be rounded to the nearest 100 mg.

PO (Children): 100–250 mg/kg/day initially, given in 2–4 divided doses immediately before meals/feedings.

Availability

Tablets: 200 mg.

NURSING IMPLICATIONS

Assessment

- Assess for hyperammonemia (neurological status, plasma ammonia levels) during therapy.
- *Lab Test Considerations:* Monitor plasma ammonia levels periodically during therapy. Maintain within normal range for age via individual dose adjustment.
- May cause ↓ hemoglobin.

Potential Nursing Diagnoses

Activity intolerance

Implementation

- Concommitant administration of other ammonia-lowering therapies is recommended.
- **PO:** Disperse each 250 mg tablet in at least 2.5 mL of water immediately before use and take immediately; do not crush or swallow whole. Tablets may not dissolve completely in water; undissolved particles may remain in mixing container. Rinse mixing container with additional volumes of water to ensure complete delivery of dose; swallow immediately. Administer via oral syringe or nasogastric tube.
- Refrigerate before opening. After first opening of container, do not refrigerate. Keep container tightly closed to protect from moisture. Write date of opening on tablet container; discard 1 month after first opening. Do not use after expiration date stated on container.

Patient/Family Teaching

- Instruct patient to take carglumic acid as directed.
- Advise patient that during acute hyperammonemic episodes, protein restriction and hypercaloric intake is recommended to block ammonia generating catabolic pathways. When plasma ammonia levels have normalized, protein intake can usually be ↑ with goal of unrestricted protein intake.
- Advise female patients to notify health care professional if pregnancy is

planned or suspected or if breastfeeding Due to risk of neurologic complications in NAGS patients, carglumic acid must be used throughout pregnancy.

Evaluation/Desired Outcomes
• Normalization of plasma ammonia levels.

---

ceftaroline
(sef-**tar**-oh-leen)
Teflaro

Classification
Thera: anti-infectives
Pharm: cephalosporins
(derivative)

Pregnancy Category B

Indications
Treatment of acute bacterial skin/skin structure infections and community-acquired pneumonia.

Action
Binds to bacterial cell wall membrane, causing cell death. **Therapeutic Effects:** Bactericidal action against susceptible bacteria. **Spectrum:** *Treatment of skin/skin structure infections*—Active against *Staphylococcus aureus* (including methicillin-susceptible and -resistant strains), *Streptococcus pyogenes, Streptococcus agalactiae, Escherichia coli, Klebsiella pneumoniae,* and *Klebsiella oxytoca; Treatment of community acquired pneumonia*—*Streptococcus pneumoniae*(including pneumonia with bacteremia), *Staphylococcus aureus*(methicillin-susceptible strains only), *Haemophilus influenzae, Klebsiella pneumoniae, Klebsiella oxytoca,* and *Escherichia coli.*

Pharmacokinetics
Absorption: IV administration results in complete bioavailability of parent drug.
Distribution: Unknown.
Metabolism and Excretion: Ceftaroline fosamil is rapidly converted by plasma phosphatases to ceftaroline, the active metabolite; 88% excreted in urine, 6% in feces.
Half-life: 2.6 hr (after multiple doses).

TIME/ACTION PROFILE (blood levels)

ROUTE	ONSET	PEAK	DURATION
IV	rapid	end of infusion	12 hr

Contraindications/Precautions
Contraindicated in: Known serious hypersensitivity to cephalosporins.
Use Cautiously in: Known hypersensitivity to other beta-lactams; Renal impairment (dosage reduction required for CCr ≤50 mL/min); Geri: dose adjustment may be necessary for age-related ↓ in renal function; OB: Use in pregnancy only if potential benefit outweighs potential risk to fetus; Lactation: Use cautiously if breastfeeding; Pedi: Safe and effective use in children <18 yr not established.

Adverse Reactions/Side Effects
GI: PSEUDOMEMBRANOUS COLITIS, diarrhea, nausea. **Derm:** rash. **Hemat:** hemolytic anemia. **Local:** phlebitis at injection site. **Misc:** hypersensitivity reactions including ANAPHYLAXIS.

Interactions
Drug-Drug: None noted.

Route/Dosage
IV (Adults 18 yr): *Skin/skin structure infections*—600 mg every 12 hr for 5–14 days; *Community-acquired pneumonia*—600 mg every 12 hr for 5–7 days.

Renal Impairment
IV (Adults >18 yr): *CCr >30 to ≤50 mL/min*—400 mg every 12 hr; *CCr ≥15 to ≤30 mL/min*—300 mg every 12 hr; *CCr <15 mL/min*—200 mg every 12 hr.

Availability
Powder for injection (requires reconstitution: 400 mg/vial, 600 mg/vial.

NURSING IMPLICATIONS

Assessment

- Assess for infection (vital signs; appearance of wound, sputum, urine, and stool; WBC) at beginning of and throughout therapy.
- Before initiating therapy, obtain a history to determine previous use of and reactions to penicillins, cephalosporins or carbapenems. Persons with a negative history of sensitivity may still have an allergic response.
- Obtain specimens for culture and sensitivity before initiating therapy. First dose may be given before receiving results.
- Observe patient for signs and symptoms of anaphylaxis (rash, pruritus, laryngeal edema, wheezing). Discontinue the drug and notify health care professional immediately if these symptoms occur. Keep epinephrine, an antihistamine, and resuscitation equipment close by in the event of an anaphylactic reaction.
- Monitor bowel function. Diarrhea, abdominal cramping, fever, and bloody stools should be reported to health care professional promptly as a sign of pseudomembranous colitis. May begin up to several mo following cessation of therapy.
- *Lab Test Considerations:* May cause seroconversion from a negative to a positive direct Coombs' test. If anemia develops during or after therapy, perform a direct Coombs' test. If drug-induced hemolytic anemia is suspected, discontinue ceftaroline and provide supportive care.

Potential Nursing Diagnoses

Risk for infection (Indications, Side Effects)

Diarrhea (Adverse Reactions)

Implementation

- **Intermittent Infusion:** Reconstitute with 20 mL of sterile water for injection. *Diluent:* Dilute further with at least 250 mL of 0.9% NaCl, D5W, D2.5W, 0.45% NaCl, or LR. Mix gently to dissolve. Solution is clear to light or dark yellow; do not administer solutions that are discolored or contain particulate matter. Solution is stable for 6 hr at room temperature or 24 hr if refrigerated. *Rate:* Infuse over 1 hr.
- **Additive Incompatibility:** Do not mix with other drugs or solutions.

Patient/Family Teaching

- Explain the purpose of ceftaroline to patient. Emphasize the importance of completing therapy, even if feeling better.
- Instruct patient to notify health care professional if fever and diarrhea develop, especially if stool contains blood, pus, or mucus. Advise patient not to treat diarrhea without consulting health care professional.

Evaluation/Desired Outcomes

- Resolution of the signs and symptoms of infection. Length of time for complete resolution depends on the organism and site of infection.

ciclesonide (inhalation)
(si-**kless**-o-nide)
Alvesco

Classification
Thera: antiasthmatics
Pharm: corticosteroids (inhalation)

Pregnancy Category C

Indications

Maintenance treatment of asthma as preventive therapy in patients ≥12 yr. Not for acute treatment of bronchospasm.

Action

Potent, locally acting anti-inflammatory and immune modifier. **Therapeutic Effects:** ↓ frequency and severity of asthma attacks; improved asthma symptoms.

Pharmacokinetics

Absorption: Negligible oral bioavailability, action is primarily local.
Distribution: Unknown.
Metabolism and Excretion: Converted by esterases to des-ciclesonide, the active drug, which is subsequently metab-

olized by the liver. Some further metabolites may be pharmacologically active. Mostly eliminated in feces via biliary excretion; <20% of des-ciclesonide is excreted in urine.

Half-life: *Ciclesonide*—0.7 hr; *Des-ciclesonide*—6–7 hr.

TIME/ACTION PROFILE (improvement in symptoms)

ROUTE	ONSET	PEAK	DURATION
Inhaln	within 24 hr	1–4 wk†	unknown

† Improvement in pulmonary function, ↓ airway responsiveness may take longer.

Contraindications/Precautions

Contraindicated in: Hypersensitivity to ciclesonide or any other ingredients in the formulation; Acute asthma/status asthmaticus.

Use Cautiously in: Geri: Consider age-related ↓ in cardiac, renal and hepatic function, concurrent disease state and drug therapy; consider lower initial dose; OB: ↓ dose may be sufficient; Lactation: Many corticosteroids enter breast milk, hypercorticism may be seen with ↑ maternal doses; Pedi: Safety and effectiveness in children <12 has not been established.

Adverse Reactions/Side Effects

CNS: headache. **EENT:** candida infection of mouth and pharynx, nasal congestion, nasopharyngitis, pharyngolaryngeal pain, cataracts, ↑ intraocular pressure. **Endo:** adrenal suppression (↑ dose, long term therapy), ↓ growth (children). **MS:** arthralgia, back pain, ↓ bone mineral density (↑ dose, long term therapy), extremity pain. **Misc:** worsening of infections.

Interactions

Drug-Drug: None noted.

Route/Dosage

Inhaln (Adults ≥12 yr): *Previous therapy with bronchodilators alone*—80 mcg twice daily, may be ↑ to 160 mcg twice daily; *Previous therapy with inhaled corticosteroids*—80 mcg twice daily, may be ↑ to 320 mcg twice daily; *Previous therapy with oral corticosteroids*—320 mcg twice daily.

Availability

Aerosol inhalation (contains HFA-134A as a propellant): 80 mcg/actuation in 6.1 g cannisters of 60 actuations, 160 mcg/actuation in 6.1 and 9.6 g cannisters of 60 and 120 actuations.

NURSING IMPLICATIONS

Assessment

- Monitor respiratory status and lung sounds. Pulmonary function tests may be assessed periodically during and for several months following a transfer from systemic to inhalation corticosteroids.

- Assess patients changing from systemic corticosteroids to inhalation corticosteroids for signs of adrenal insufficiency (anorexia, nausea, weakness, fatigue, hypotension, hypoglycemia) during initial therapy and periods of stress. If these signs appear, notify health care professional immediately; condition may be life-threatening.

- Monitor for withdrawal symptoms (fatigue, weakness, nausea, vomiting, hypotension, joint or muscular pain, lassitude, depression) during withdrawal from oral corticosteroids.

- Monitor growth rates in children receiving chronic therapy; lowest possible dose should be used.

- Monitor patients with a change in vision or with a history of ↑ intraocular pressure, glaucoma, or cataracts closely.

- *Lab Test Considerations:* Periodic adrenal function tests may be ordered to assess degree of hypothalamic-pituitary-adrenal (HPA) axis suppression in chronic therapy. Children and patients using higher than recommended doses are at highest risk for HPA suppression.

Potential Nursing Diagnoses

Ineffective airway clearance (Indications)
Risk for infection (Side Effects)

Implementation

- When changing from oral to inhaled corticosteroids, taper oral dose slowly, no faster than prednisone 2.5 mg/day on a weekly basis, beginning after at least 1 wk of ciclesonide inhalation therapy.

- After the desired clinical effect has been obtained, attempts should be made to ↓ dose to lowest amount required to control symptoms. Gradually ↓ as long as desired effect is maintained. If symptoms return, dose may briefly return to starting dose.
- **Inhaln:** Allow at least 1 min between inhalations. Do not shake inhaler or use with spacer (See Appendix D).
- If bronchospasm occurs right after ciclesonide dose, discontinue and administer short acting bronchodilator; notify health care professional.

Patient/Family Teaching

- Instruct patient to use inhaler at regular intervals as directed. If a dose is missed, omit and take next regularly scheduled dose. Advise patient not to ↑ dose or discontinue medication, even if feeling better, without consulting health care professional; gradual ↓ is required. If asthma symptoms worsen, contact health care professional. Instruct patient to read *Patient Leaflet* before use.
- Advise patient to follow instructions supplied. Before first-time use or if inhaler has not been used for more than 10 days, prime unit by actuating 3 times prior to dose. Do not shake inhaler. When dose indicator display window shows a red zone, 20 inhalations are left and refill is required; discard when indicator shows zero. Do not use actuator with other medications. Clean mouthpiece weekly with a clean dry tissue; do not wash or put any part of the inhaler in water.
- Advise patients using inhalation corticosteroids and bronchodilator to use bronchodilator first and to allow 5 min to elapse before administering the corticosteroid, unless otherwise directed by health care professional.
- Advise patient that inhalation corticosteroids should not be used to treat an acute asthma attack but should be continued even if other inhalation agents are used.
- Instruct patient to notify health care professional if asthma worsens or if signs of adrenal insufficiency occur.
- Patients using inhalation corticosteroids to control asthma may require systemic corticosteroids for acute attacks. Advise patient to use regular peak flow monitoring to determine respiratory status.
- Advise patient to rinse mouth with water after treatment to ↓ risk of developing local candidiasis.
- Caution patient to avoid smoking, known allergens, and other respiratory irritants.
- Advise patient to notify health care professional if sore throat or mouth occurs or if exposed to anyone with chicken pox or measles.
- Instruct patient to consult health care professional before taking other Rx, OTC, or herbal products.
- Advise female patients to notify health care professional if pregnancy is planned or suspected or if breastfeeding.
- Instruct patient whose systemic corticosteroids have been recently reduced or withdrawn to carry a warning card indicating the need for supplemental systemic corticosteroids in the event of stress or severe asthma attack unresponsive to bronchodilators.

Evaluation/Desired Outcomes

- Management of the symptoms of chronic asthma.
- Improvement in asthma symptoms. Maximum benefit may take 4 wks or longer.

---

collagenase clostridium histolyticum

(kol-**la**-jen-ase kloss-**trid**-ee-yum **his**-toe-**lit**-i-cum)

Xiaflex

Classification

Thera: none assigned

Pregnancy Category B

Indications

Treatment of Dupuytren's contracture with a palpable cord in adults.

Action

Lysis of collagen deposits present in Dupuytren's cord. **Therapeutic Effects:** Enzymatic disruption of Dupuytren's cord.

Pharmacokinetics

Absorption: Unknown.
Distribution: Unknown.
Metabolism and Excretion: Unknown.
Half-life: Unknown.

TIME/ACTION PROFILE (cord disruption)

ROUTE	ONSET	PEAK	DURATION
Intralesional	within 24 hr	unknown	unknown

Contraindications/Precautions

Contraindicated in: None known.
Use Cautiously in: Abnormal coagulation, including concurrent anticoagulants other than low-dose aspirin within 7 days of treatment; OB: Use during pregnancy only if clearly needed; Lactation: Use cautiously during lactation; Pedi: Safety and effectiveness in children <18 yr not established.

Adverse Reactions/Side Effects

CV: vasovagal syncope. **MS:** ligament injury, complex regional pain syndrome (CRPS), sensory abnormality of hand, tendon rupture. **Local:** contusion, hemorrhage, injection site reaction, pain, pruritus, swelling. **Misc:** allergic reactions including ANAPHYLAXIS, axillary pain, lymphadenopathy.

Interactions

Drug-Drug: Concurrent use of **anticoagulants** may ↑ risk of local bleeding.

Route/Dosage

IL (Adults): 0.58 mg into a palpable cord with a contracture of a metacarpophalangeal (MP) joint or a proximal interphalangeal (PIP) joint.

Availability

Lyophilized powder for injection (requires reconstitution): 0.9 mg/vial (delivers 0.58 mg/dose).

NURSING IMPLICATIONS

Assessment

● Assess severity of Dupuytren's contracture prior to and following injection.

Potential Nursing Diagnoses

Impaired physical mobility (Indications)
Acute pain (Adverse Reactions)

Implementation

● Allow powder and diluent vials to stand at room temperature for 15–60 min prior to mixing. Use only diluent supplied for reconstitution. Use a syringe with 0.01 mL graduations with a 27 gauge, 1/2 inch needle to withdraw diluent. Withdraw 0.39 mL for cords affecting a MP joint and 0.31 mL for cords affecting a PIP joint. Inject diluent slowly into sides of vial; do not invert of shake vial. Slowly swirl solution to ensure all powder is in solution. Reconstituted solution should be clear without particulate matter. Solution is stable for 1 hr at room temperature or up to 4 hrs if refrigerated. If refrigerated, allow to stand at room temperature for 15 min before administering.

● **IL:** Do not administer local anesthesia prior to injection; may interfere with placement of medication. Use a new hubless syringe with 0.01 graduations with a permanently fixed, 27-gauge, 1/2 inch needle to withdraw volume to be injected. For MP joint, withdraw 0.25 mL. For PIP joint, withdraw 0.20 mL. Follow manufacturer's instructions for injection procedure.

● Wrap hand with a bulky dressing following injection.

Patient/Family Teaching

● Instruct patient to return to health care professional's office the next day for an examination of the injected hand and for possible finger extension procedure to disrupt the cord.

- Instruct patient not to flex fingers of injected hand to reduce extravasation of medication out of the cord.
- Advise patient not to disrupt injected cord by manipulation.
- Instruct patient to elevate hand as much as possible until bedtime.
- Advise patient that injection is likely to result in swelling, bruising, bleeding, and/or pain of the injected site and surrounding tissue.
- Advise patient to promptly notify health care professional if signs of infection (fever, chills, increasing redness or swelling), sensory changes in the treated finger, trouble bending the finger after swelling goes down occur.

Evaluation/Desired Outcomes
- Reduction in Dupuytren's contracture.

---

dabigatran
(da-bye-**gat**-ran)
Pradaxa

Classification
Thera: anticoagulants
Pharm: thrombin inhibitors

Pregnancy Category C

Indications
To ↓ risk of stroke/systemic embolization associated with non-valvular atrial fibrillation.

Action
Acts as a direct inhibitor of thrombin.
Therapeutic Effects: Lowered risk of thrombotic sequelae (stroke and systemic embolization) of non-valvular atrial fibrillation.

Pharmacokinetics
Absorption: 3–7% absorbed following oral administration.
Distribution: Unknown.
Metabolism and Excretion: Of the amount absorbed, mostly excreted by kidneys (80%); 86% of ingested dose is eliminated in feces due to poor bioavailability.
Half-life: 12–17 hr.

TIME/ACTION PROFILE (effects on coagulation)

ROUTE	ONSET	PEAK	DURATION
PO	within hours	unknown	2 days†

†Following discontinuation, 3–5 days in renal impairment.

Contraindications/Precautions
Contraindicated in: Hypersensitivity; Active pathological bleeding; Concurrent use of Pg-P inducers.
Use Cautiously in: Concurrent medications/pre-existing conditions that ↑ bleeding risk (other anticoagulants, antiplatelet agents, antifibrinolytics, heparins, chronic NSAID use, labor and delivery); Surgical procedures (discontinue 1–2 days prior if CCr ≥50 mL/min or 3–4 days prior if CCr <50 mL/min; Geri: ↑ risk of bleeding; Lactation: Use cautiously during breastfeeding; Pedi: Safety and effectiveness not established.

Adverse Reactions/Side Effects
GI: abdominal pain, diarrhea, dyspepsia, gastritis, nausea. **Hemat:** BLEEDING.
Misc: hypersensitivity reactions including ANAPHYLAXIS.

Interactions
Drug-Drug: Concurrent use of other **anticoagulants**, **antiplatelet agents**, **antifibrinolytics**, **heparins**, **prasugrel**, **clopidogrel**, or chronic use of **NSAIDs** ↑ risk of bleeding. Concurrent use of **P-gp inducers** including **rifampin** ↓ blood levels and effectiveness and should be avoided.

Route/Dosage
PO (Adults): 150 mg twice daily; *CCr 15–30 mL/min*—75 mg twice daily.

Availability
Capsules: 75 mg, 150 mg.

NURSING IMPLICATIONS
Assessment
- Assess patient for symptoms of stroke or peripheral vascular disease periodically during therapy.

Potential Nursing Diagnoses
Activity intolerance

Implementation

- When *converting from warfarin*, discontinue warfarin and start dabigatran when INR is <2.0.
- When *converting from dabigatran to warfarin*, adjust starting time based on creatinine clearance. For *CCr >50 mL/min*, start warfarin 3 days before discontinuing dabigatran. For *CCr 31–50 mL/min*, start warfarin 2 days before discontinuing dabigatran. For *CCr 15–30 mL/min*, start warfarin 1 day before discontinuing dabigatran. For *CCr <15 mL/min*, no recommendations can be made. INR will better reflect warfarin's effect after dabigatran has been stopped for at least 2 days.
- When *converting from parenteral anticoagulants*, start dabigatran up to 2 hrs before next dose of parenteral drug is due or at time of discontinuation of parenteral therapy.
- When *converting to dabigatran from parenteral anticoagulants*, wait 12 hrs (CCr ≥30 mL/min) or 24 hr (CCr <30 mL/min) after last dose of dabigatran before initiating parenteral anticoagulant therapy.
- *For surgery*, discontinue dabigatran 1–2 days (CrCL ≥50 mL/min) or 3–5 days (CCr <50 mL/min) before invasive or surgical procedures; consider longer times for major surgery, spinal puncture, or placement of a spinal or epidural catheter. If surgery cannot be delayed, bleeding risk is ↑. Assess bleeding risk with ecarin clotting time (ECT) or aPTT is ECT is not available.
- **PO:** Administer twice daily without regard to food. Swallow capsule whole; do not open, crush, or chew.

Patient/Family Teaching

- Instruct patient to take dabigatran as directed. Do not discontinue without consulting health care professional, If temporarily discontinued, restart as soon as possible.
- Inform patient that they may bleed more easily or longer than usual. Advise patient to notify health care professional

immediately if signs of bleeding (unusual bruising, pink or brown urine, red or black, tarry stools, coughing up blood, vomiting blood, pain or swelling in a joint, headache, dizziness, weakness, recurring nose bleeds, unusual bleeding from gums, heavier than normal menstrual bleeding, dyspepsia, abdominal pain, epigastric pain) occurs.
- Advise patient to notify health care professional of medication regimen prior to treatment or surgery.
- Instruct patient to notify health care professional of all Rx or OTC medications, vitamins, or herbal products being taken and consult health care professional before taking any new medications.
- Advise female patient to notify health care professional if pregnancy is planned or suspected or if breastfeeding.

Evaluation/Desired Outcomes

- Reduction in the risk of stroke and systemic embolism.

---

dalfampridine
(dal-**fam**-pri-deen)
Ampyra, 4-aminopyridine, 4-AP, fampridine

Classification
Thera: anti-multiple sclerosis agents
Pharm: potassium channel blocker

Pregnancy Category C

Indications
Treatment of mutiple sclerosis, to improve walking speed.

Action
Acts as a potassium channel blocker, which may ↑ conduction of action potentials. **Therapeutic Effects:** ↑ walking speed in patients with multiple sclerosis.

✦ = Canadian drug name. ☒ = Genetic implication.
*CAPITALS indicates life-threatening; underlines indicate most frequent.

Pharmacokinetics

Absorption: Rapidly and completely absorbed (96%).
Distribution: Unknown.
Metabolism and Excretion: 96% eliminated in urine, 0.5% in feces.
Half-life: 5.2–6.5 hr.

TIME/ACTION PROFILE (improvement in walking speed)

ROUTE	ONSET	PEAK	DURATION
PO	unknown	3–4 hr	24 hr

Contraindications/Precautions

Contraindicated in: History of seizures; Moderate/severe renal impairment (↑ risk of seizures); Lactation: Avoid use during lactation.
Use Cautiously in: Geri: Consider age-related ↓ in renal function; OB: Use during pregnancy only if potential benefit justifies potential risk to fetus; Pedi: safety and effectiveness in children <18 yr not established.

Adverse Reactions/Side Effects

CNS: SEIZURES, dizziness, headache, insomnia, weakness. **EENT:** nasopharyngitis, pharyngolaryngeal pain. **GI:** constipation, dyspepsia, nausea. **GU:** urinary tract infection. **MS:** back pain. **Neuro:** balance disorder, muliple sclerosis relapse, paresthesia.

Interactions

Drug-Drug: None noted.

Route/Dosage

PO (Adults): 10 mg twice daily.

Availability

Extended-release tablets: 10 mg.

NURSING IMPLICATIONS

Assessment

● Assess walking speed in patients with multiple sclerosis prior to and periodically during therapy.
● Monitor for seizures during therapy, risk ↑s with ↑ dose. If seizure occurs, discontinue therapy.

Potential Nursing Diagnoses

Impaired walking (Indications)

Implementation

● Administer tablets twice daily approximately 12 hrs apart without regard to food. Administer tablets whole; do not break, crush, chew or dissolve.

Patient/Family Teaching

● Instruct patient to take dalfampridine as directed, with approximately 12 hrs between tablets. If a dose is missed, omit and take next scheduled dose on time; do not double doses. May ↑ risk of seizures.
● Advise patient to tell health care professional what medications they are taking and to avoid taking new Rx, OTC, vitamins, or herbal products without consulting health care professional.
● Advise female patient to notify health care professional if pregnancy is planned or suspected or if breastfeeding.

Evaluation/Desired Outcomes

● Improved walking and ↑ walking speed in patients with multiple sclerosis.

denosumab
(de-**no**-su-mab)
Prolia

Classification
Thera: bone resorption inhibitors
Pharm: monoclonal antibodies

Pregnancy Category C

Indications

Treatment of osteoporosis postmenopausal women who are at high risk for fracture or those who have failed/are intolerant of conventional osteoporosis therapy.

Action

A monoclonal antibody that binds specifically to the human receptor activator of nuclear factor kappa-B-ligand (RANKL), which is required for formation, function and survival of osteoclasts. Binding inhibits osteoclast formation, function and survival. **Therapeutic Effects:** ↓ bone resorption with ↓ occurrence of fractures (vertebral, nonvertebral, hip).

Pharmacokinetics
Absorption: Well absorbed following subcutaneous administration.
Distribution: Unknown.
Metabolism and Excretion: Unknown.
Half-life: 25.4 days.

TIME/ACTION PROFILE (effects on bone resorption)

ROUTE	ONSET	PEAK	DURATION
Subcut	1 mo	unknown†	12 mo‡

†Maximum ↓ in serum calcium occurs at 10 days.
‡Following discontinuation.

Contraindications/Precautions
Contraindicated in: Hypocalcemia (correct before administering); adequate supplemental calcium and Vitamin D required; Lactation: Avoid use; ↓ s mammary gland development and lactation.
Use Cautiously in: Conditions associated with hypocalcemia including hypoparathyroidism, previous thyroid/parathyroid surgery, malabsorption syndromes, history of small intestinal excision, renal impairment/hemodialysis (CCr <30 mL/min); monitoring of calcium and other minerals recommended; Concurrent use of immunosuppressants or diseases resulting in immunosuppression (↑ risk of infection); Geri: May be more sensitive to drug effects; OB: Use in pregnancy only when potential benefit justifies potential risk to fetus; Pedi: Safe and effective use not established.

Adverse Reactions/Side Effects
GI: PANCREATITIS. **GU:** cystitis. **Derm:** dermatitis, eczema, rashes. **F and E:** hypocalcemia. **Metab:** hypercholesterolemia. **MS:** back pain, extremity pain, musculoskeletal pain, osteonecrosis of the jaw, suppression of bone turnover. **Misc:** infection.

Interactions
Drug-Drug: Concurrent use of **immunosuppressants** ↑ risk of infection.

Route/Dosage
Subcut (Adults females): 60 mg every six mo.

Availability
Solution for injection: 60 mg/ 1 mL in 1–mL prefilled syringes and vials.

NURSING IMPLICATIONS
Assessment
- Assess patients via bone density study for low bone mass before and periodically during therapy.
- Perform a routine oral exam prior to initiation of therapy. Dental exam with appropriate preventative dentistry should be considered prior to therapy.
- *Lab Test Considerations:* Assess serum calcium, phosphorous and magnesium levels before and periodically during therapy. Hypocalcemia and vitamin D deficiency should be treated before initiating therapy. May cause mild, transient ↑ of calcium and phosphate.
- May cause anemia.
- May cause hypercholesterolemia.

Potential Nursing Diagnoses
Risk for injury (Indications)

Implementation
- Grey needle cap on single-use pre-filled syringe should not be handled by people sensitive to latex.
- **Subcut:** May remove from refrigerator and bring to room temperature by standing in original container for 15–30 min prior to administration; do not warm in any other way. Do not shake. Administer in the upper arm, upper thigh, or abdomen. Solution is clear and colorless to pale yellow, and may contain trace amounts of translucent to white proteinaceous particles. Do not use if solution is discolored or contains many particles. Manually activate the green safety guard *after* the injection is given, not before.

✢ = Canadian drug name. ⚇ = Genetic implication.
*CAPITALS indicates life-threatening; underlines indicate most frequent.

- Patients should receive calcium 1000 mg and 400 IU vitamin D daily.

Patient/Family Teaching

- Explain the purpose of denosumab to patient. If a dose is missed, administer injection as soon as possible; schedule injections every 6 mo from date of last injection.
- Advise patient to eat a balanced diet and consult health care professional about the need for supplemental calcium and vitamin D (see Appendix M).
- Advise patient to notify health professional immediately if signs of hypocalcemia (spasms, twitches, or cramps in muscles; numbness or tingling in fingers, toes, or around mouth), infection (fever, chills, skin that is red, swollen, hot, or tender to touch; severe abdominal pain, frequent or urgent need to urinate or burning during urination), or skin reactions (redness, itching, rash, dry or leathery feeling, blisters that ooze or become crusty, peeling) occur.
- Encourage patient to participate in regular exercise and to modify behaviors that ↑ the risk of osteoporosis (stop smoking, reduce alcohol consumption).
- Advise patient to take good care of teeth and gums (brush and floss regularly) and to inform health care professional of therapy prior to dental surgery.
- Advise female patients to notify health care professional if pregnancy is planned or suspected or if breastfeeding.

Evaluation/Desired Outcomes

- Reversal of the progression of osteoporosis with ↓ fractures and other sequelae.

ecallantide
(ee-**kal**-lan-tide)
Kalbitor

Classification
Thera: antiangioedema agents
Pharm: kallikrein inhibitors

Pregnancy Category C

Indications
Treatment of acute attacks of hereditary angioedema (HAE) in patients ≥16 yr.

Action
Acts as a selective, reversible inhibitor of kallikrein, thereby inhibiting its action in initiating bradykinin production, part of the cascade of events in hereditary angioedema (HAE). **Therapeutic Effects:** ↓ severity of attack of HAE.

Pharmacokinetics
Absorption: Well absorbed following subcutaneous administration.
Distribution: Unknown.
Metabolism and Excretion: Renally eliminated.
Half-life: 2 hr.

TIME/ACTION PROFILE (symptom improvement)

ROUTE	ONSET	PEAK	DURATION
SC	unknown	2–4 hr	up to 24 hr

Contraindications/Precautions
Contraindicated in: Known hypersensitivity.
Use Cautiously in: Geri: Consider age-related ↓ in hepatic, renal, or cardiac function, concomitant diseases or other drug therapy; lower initial dose may be considered; Lactation: Use cautiously; OB: Use during pregnancy only if clearly needed.

Adverse Reactions/Side Effects
CNS: headache, fatigue. **EENT:** nasopharyngitis. **GI:** nausea, abdominal pain, diarrhea. **Derm:** pruritus, rash, urticaria. **Local:** injection site reactions. **Misc:** allergic reactions including ANAPHYLAXIS, fever.

Interactions
Drug-Drug: None noted.

Route/Dosage
Subcut (Adults ≥16 yr): 30 mg given as three 10 mg injections; an additional dose of 30 mg may be given within 24 hr.

Availability
Injection for subcutaneous use: 10 mg/mL in 1-mL vials.

NURSING IMPLICATIONS

Assessment
- Assess for symptoms of hereditary angioedema (submucosal or subcutaneous swelling) before and following treatment.
- Assess for signs and symptoms of anaphylaxis (chest discomfort, flushing, pharyngeal edema, pruritus, rhinorrhea, sneezing, nasal congestion, throat irritation, urticaria, wheezing, hypotension); usually occur within 1 hr of administration.

Potential Nursing Diagnoses
Ineffective breathing pattern (Adverse Reactions)

Implementation
- **Subcut:** Use a large bore needle to withdraw ecallantide from vial. Change needles. Solution should be clear and colorless; do not administer solutions that are discolored or contain a precipitate. Administer three 1 mL (10 mg/mL) injections using a 27 gauge needle into abdomen, thigh, or upper arm for a total dose of 30 mg. Injection site for each of the 3 injections may be in the same or different locations; no need for rotation. Separate injection sites by at least 2 inches from site of angioedema attack. If attack persists, may repeat dose, using same instructions, within 24 hrs.

Patient/Family Teaching
- Instruct patient in the purpose for ecallantide and the need for administration by health care professional. Advise patient to read *Medication Guide* prior to administration.
- Caution patient of the risk for anaphylactic reaction usually within 1 hr of injection. Advise patient to notify health care professional immediately if signs and symptoms of anaphylactic reactions occur.
- Inform patient that injection site reactions (local pruritus, erythema, pain, irritation, uriticaria, bruising) may occur.
- Advise patient to notify health care professional of Rx, OTC, vitamins, and herbal products being taken.
- Advise female patients to notify health care professional if pregnancy is planned or suspected or if breastfeeding.

Evaluation/Desired Outcomes
- Resolution of signs and symptoms of an acute attack of hereditary angioedema.

---

eribulin (e-rib-yoo-lin)
Halaven

Classification
Thera: antineoplastics
Pharm: microtubule inhibitors

Pregnancy Category D

Indications
Metastatic breast cancer that has progressed despite at least two previous regimens which included an anthracycline and a taxane in either regimen.

Action
Inhibits intracellular microtubule growth phase, causing G_2/M cell-cycle block resulting in apoptotic cell death. **Therapeutic Effects:** Death of rapidly replicating cells, particularly malignant ones. ↓ spread of breast cancer.

Pharmacokinetics
Absorption: IV administration results in complete bioavailability.
Distribution: Unknown.
Metabolism and Excretion: Minimal metabolism, mostly excreted unchanged in feces (82%) and less in urine (9%).
Half-life: 40 hr.

TIME/ACTION PROFILE (effects on blood counts)

ROUTE	ONSET	PEAK	DURATION
IV	within days	7–14 days	up to 2 wk

Contraindications/Precautions

Contraindicated in: Severe hepatic impairment; Severe renal impairment (CCr <30mL/min); Congenital long QT syndrome; OB: Pregnancy; may cause fetal harm; Lactation: Avoid breastfeeding.
Use Cautiously in: CHF, bradyarrhythmias, concurrent use of drugs known to prolong the QT interval (including Class Ia and III antiarrhythmics), electrolyte abnormalities (↑ risk of arrhythmias); Moderate renal impairment; lower initial dose recommended for CCr 30–50 mL/min; Mild to moderate hepatic impairment; lower initial dose recommended; OB: Women with childbearing potential; Pedi: Safe and effective use in children <18 yr has not been established.

Adverse Reactions/Side Effects

CNS: fatigue, weakness, depression, dizziness, headache, insomnia. **EENT:** ↑ lacrimation. **CV:** QTc PROLONGATION, peripheral edema. **Resp:** cough, dyspnea, upper respiratory tract infection. **GI:** anorexia, constipation, nausea, abdominal pain, abnormal taste, dry mouth, dyspepsia, mucositis, diarrhea, vomiting. **Derm:** alopecia, rash. **F and E:** hypokalemia. **Hemat:** ANEMIA, NEUTROPENIA. **MS:** arthralgia, myalgia. **Neuro:** peripheral neuropathy. **Misc:** fever, urinary tract infection.

Interactions

Drug-Drug: ↑ risk of bone marrow depression with other **antineoplastics** or **radiation therapy**. ↓ antibody response and ↑ risk of adverse reactions with **live virus vaccines**.

Route/Dosage

IV (Adults): 1.4 mg/m² on days 1 and 8 of a 21 day cycle; dose modifications required for hepatic impairment, moderate renal impairment, neutropenia, thrombocytopenia, or peripheral neuropathy.

Renal Impairment

IV (Adults): *Mild hepatic impairment (Child-Pugh A)* — 1.1 mg/m² on days 1 and 8 of a 21 day cycle *Moderate hepatic impairment (Child-Pugh B)* — 0.7 mg/m² on days 1 and 8 of a 21 day cycle.

Renal Impairment

IV (Adults): *Moderate renal impairment (CCr 30–50 mL/min)* — 1.1 mg/m² on days 1 and 8 of a 21 day cycle.

Availability

Solution for IV administration: 0.5 mg/mL in 2-mL vials.

NURSING IMPLICATIONS

Assessment

- Assess for peripheral motor and sensory neuropathy (numbness, tingling, burning in hands or feet). Withhold eribulin in patients who experience Grade 3 or 4 peripheral neuropathy until resolution to Grade 2 or less.
- Monitor ECG periodically as indicated.
- *Lab Test Considerations:* Monitor CBC prior to each dose; ↑ frequency of monitoring in patients who develop Grade 3 or 4 cytopenias. Delay administration and reduce subsequent doses in patients who develop febrile neutropenia or Grade 4 neutropenia lasting longer than 7 days.
- Monitor electrolytes periodically during therapy.

Potential Nursing Diagnoses

Activity intolerance

Implementation

- Correct hypokalemia or hypomagnesemia prior to initiating therapy.

IV Administration

- *Do not administer on Day 1 or Day 8 if:* ANC <1000/mm³, platelets <75,000/mm³, or Grade 3 or 4 non-hematological toxicities occur.
- *Day 8 dose may be delayed for a maximum of 1 wk:* If toxicities do not resolve or improve to ≤Grade 2 severity by Day 15, omit dose.
- If toxicities resolve or improve to ≤Grade 2 by Day 15, administer eribulin at a reduced dose and initiate next cycle no sooner than 2 wks later.
- If a dose has been delayed for toxicity and toxicities have recovered to Grade 2

severity or less, resume eribulin at a reduced dose of 1.1 mg/m².
- *Permanently reduce 1.4 mg/m² eribulin dose to 1.1 mg/m² if:* ANC <500/mm³ for >7 days, ANC <1000/mm³ either fever or infection, platelets <25,000/mm³, platelets <50,000/mm³ requiring transfusion, non-hematologic Grade 3 or 4 toxicities, or omission or delay of Day 8 eribulin dose in previous cycle for toxicity.
- *Permanently reduce 1.4 mg/m² eribulin dose to 0.7 mg/m² if:* occurrence of any event requiring permanent dose reduction while receiving 1.1 mg/m² dose.
- *If occurrence of any event requiring permanent dose reduction while receiving 0.7 mg/m²:* discontinue eribulin.
- **Direct IV: *Diluent:*** Administer undiluted or dilute in 100 mL of 0.9% NaCl. Store undiluted in syringe or diluted eribulin for up to 4 hr at room temperature or for up to 24 hr under refrigeration. Discard unused portion of vial. ***Rate:*** Infuse over 2–5 minutes on Days 1 and 8 of a 21-day cycle.
- **Y-Site Incompatibility:** Do not dilute in or administer through an IV line containing solutions with dextrose or other medications.

Patient/Family Teaching
- Advise patient to notify health care professional if fever of ≥100.5° F or other signs or symptoms of infection (chills, cough, burning or pain on urination) occur.
- Advise female patient to use effective contraception during therapy and to notify health care professional immediately if pregnancy is planned or suspected or if breastfeeding.
- Instruct patient to notify health care professional of all Rx or OTC medications, vitamins, or herbal products being taken and consult health care professional before taking any new medications.

- Advise patient not to receive vaccinations without consulting health care professional.

Evaluation/Desired Outcomes
- ↓ spread of breast cancer.

---

everolimus
(e-ve-**ro**-li-mus)
Afinitor

Classification
Thera: antineoplastics
Pharm: kinase inhibitors

Pregnancy Category D

Indications
Advanced renal cell carcinoma which has failed treatment with sunitinib or sorafenib.

Action
Acts as a kinase inhibitor, decreasing cell proliferation. **Therapeutic Effects:** ↓ spread of renal cell carcinoma.

Pharmacokinetics
Absorption: Well absorbed following oral administration.
Distribution: 20% confined to plasma.
Metabolism and Excretion: Mostly metabolized by liver and other systems (CYP3A4 and PgP; metabolites are mostly excreted in feces [80%] and urine [5%]).
Half-life: 30 hr.

TIME/ACTION PROFILE (blood levels))

ROUTE	ONSET	PEAK	DURATION
PO	unknown	1–2 hr	24 hr

Contraindications/Precautions
Contraindicated in: Hypersensitivity to everolimus or other rapamycins; Severe hepatic impairment (Child-Pugh class C); OB: May cause fetal harm, avoid use during pregnancy; Lactation: Avoid breastfeeding.
Use Cautiously in: Moderate hepatic impairment (Child-Pugh class B); dose re-

duction required; **Geri:** Elderly patients may be more sensitive to drug effects; consider age-related ↓ in hepatic function, concurrent disease states and drug therapy; **Pedi:** Safe use in children has not been established.

Adverse Reactions/Side Effects

CNS: fatigue, weakness, headache. **Resp:** PNEUMONITIS, cough, dyspnea. **GI:** anorexia, diarrhea, mucositis, mouth ulcers, nausea, stomatitis, vomiting, dysgeusia. **F and E:** peripheral edema. **Derm:** dry skin, pruritus, rash. **Hemat:** anemia, leukopenia, thrombocytopenia. **Metab:** hyperglycemia, hyperlipidemia, hypertriglyceridemia. **MS:** extremity pain. **Misc:** INFECTIONS, hypersensitivity reactions including ANAPHYLAXIS, fever.

Interactions

Drug-Drug: ↑ blood levels and risk of toxicity with moderate and strong inhibitors of **CYP 3A4 enzyme system** and **PgP** including **amprenavir, aprepitant, atazanvir, clarithromyin, delavirdine, diltiazemerythromycin, fluconazole, fosamprenavir, indinavir, itraconazole, ketoconazole, nefazodine, nelfinavir, ritonavir, saquinavir, telithromycin, verapamil,** and **voriconazole**; avoid concurrent use. Avoid concurrent use with **CYP3A4 inducers** including **carbamazepine, dexamethasone, phenobarbital, phenytoin, rifabutin,** and **rifampin;** ↑ dose of everolimus may be required. May ↓ antibody formation and ↑ risk of adverse reactions from **live virus vaccines**.

Natural-Food: ↑ blood levels and risk of toxicity with **grapefruit juice**; avoid concurrent use.

Route/Dosage

PO (Adults): 10 mg once daily; *Concurrent use of strong inducers of CYP3A4*— ↑ dose in 5 mg increments up to 20 mg/daily.

Hepatic Impairment

PO (Adults): *Moderate hepatic impairment*—5 mg once daily.

Availability

Tablets: 5 mg, 10 mg.

NURSING IMPLICATIONS

Assessment

● Assess for symptoms of non-infectious pneumonitis (hypoxia, pleural effusion, cough, dyspnea) during therapy. If symptoms are mild, therapy may continue. Therapy should be interrupted for moderate symptoms and corticosteroids may be used. Re-inititate everolimus at a reduced dose of 5 mg/day when symptoms resolve.

● Assess for mouth ulcers, stomatitis, or oral mucositis. Topical treatments may be used; avoid peroxide-containing mouthwashes and antifungals unless fungal infection has been diagnosed.

● *Lab Test Considerations:* Monitor renal function prior to and periodically during therapy. May cause ↑ BUN and serum creatinine.

● Monitor fasting serum glucose and lipid profile prior to and periodically during therapy. May cause ↑ cholesterol, triglycerides, glucose. Attempt to achieve optimal glucose and lipid control prior to therapy.

● Monitor CBC prior to and periodically during therapy; may cause ↓ hemoglobin, lymphocyte, neutrophils, and platelets.

● May cause ↑ AST, ALT, phosphate, and bilirubin.

Potential Nursing Diagnoses

Risk for infection (Adverse Reactions)

Implementation

● **PO:** Administer without regard to food, followed by a whole glass of water. Tablets should be swallowed whole; do not break, crush, or chew. Avoid grapefruit juice and grapefruit products during therapy.

Patient/Family Teaching

● Instruct patient to take everolimus at the same time each day as directed. Take missed doses as soon as remembered up to 6 hr after time of normal dose. If more than 6 hr after normal dose, omit dose for that day and take next dose next day; do not take 2 doses to make up missed dose. Do not eat grapefruit or drink grapefruit juice during therapy. Advise patient to read *Patient Information Leaflet* prior to beginning therapy and with each Rx refill in case of new information.

- Advise patient to report worsening respiratory symptoms or signs of infection to health care professional promptly.
- Inform patient that mouth sores may occur. Consult health care professional for treatment if pain, discomfort, or open sores in mouth occur. May require special mouthwash or gel.
- Instruct patient to avoid use of live vaccines and close contact with those who have received live vaccines.
- Advise patient to consult health care professional before taking any Rx, OTC, or herbal products.
- May have teratogenic effects and ↓ male and female fertility. Advise female patients to use effective contraception during and for up to 8 wks following therapy and to notify health care professional if pregnancy is planned or suspected or if breastfeeding.
- Emphasize the importance of routine blood tests to determine effectiveness and side effects.

Evaluation/Desired Outcomes

- ↓ spread of renal carcinoma. Continue treatment as long as clinical benefit is observed or until unacceptable toxicity occurs.

---

factor XIII concentrate, human (FXIII) concentrate (Human)
(fak-tor thir-teen)
Corifact

Classification
Thera: replacement clotting factors
Pharm: blood products

Pregnancy Category C

Indications
Routine preventive treatment of congenital Factor XIII deficiency.

Action
Factor XIII is a calcium- and thrombin-activated proenzyme. Once activated it catalyzes cross-linking of fibrin resulting in stabilization and resistance to fibrinolysis. Also prevents degradation of fibrin clot by plasmin; result is clot stabilization. **Therapeutic Effects:** Replaces deficient Factor XIII thereby preventing bleeding in congenital deficiency.

Pharmacokinetics
Absorption: IV administration results in complete bioavailability.
Distribution: Unknown.
Metabolism and Excretion: Unknown.
Half-life: 6 days.

TIME/ACTION PROFILE (hemostatic effect)

ROUTE	ONSET	PEAK	DURATION
IV	rapid	end of infusion	28 days

Contraindications/Precautions
Contraindicated in: Known severe hypersensitivity reactions to human plasma-derived products or any other components in the product.
Use Cautiously in: OB: Use during pregnancy only if clearly needed; pregnancy is associated ↑ risk of thrombosis; Lactation: Use only if clearly needed.

Adverse Reactions/Side Effects
CNS: headache. **EENT:** epistaxis. **GI:** abdominal pain, diarrhea, ↑ liver enzymes, vomiting. **Derm:** bruising, rash. **Hemat:** EMBOLISM, THROMBOSIS. **MS:** arthralgia, joint/limb injury. **Misc:** allergic reactions including ANAPHYLAXIS, antibody formation, fever, flu-like syndrome.

Interactions
Drug-Drug: None noted.

Route/Dosage
IV (Adults and Children): 40 units/kg, subsequent doses given every 28 days de-

termined to maintain a trough FXIII level of 5–20%.

Availability

Concentrate for IV infusion (requires reconstitution and further dilution): 1000–1600 units/vial.

NURSING IMPLICATIONS

Assessment

- Monitor for hypersensitivity reactions (allergy, rash, pruritus, erythema, urticaria, chest tightness, wheezing, hypotension). If signs occur, discontinue infusion and institute appropriate treatment. Pyrogenic reactions (fever, chills) may also occur.
- Monitor for development of inhibitory antibodies. May manifest as inadequate response to treatment or breakthrough bleeding during prophylaxis. If suspected, perform an assay that measures FXIII inhibitory antibody concentrations.
- *Lab Test Considerations:* Monitor trough FXIII activity levels with each treatment.

Potential Nursing Diagnoses

Ineffective tissue perfusion (Indications)

Implementation

- Dose is based on the most recent trough. If trough level is < 5%, ↑ dose by 5 units/kg, if trough level is 5–20% continue with 40 units/kg dose; if two trough levels >20% or one trough level >25% ↓ dose by 5 units/kg.
- Record the batch number of the product in the medical record every with each administration.

IV Administration

- **Direct IV:** Ensure vial is at room temperature. Do not use beyond expiration date. Reconstitute Mix2Vial as directed by manufacturer. Solution is colorless to slightly yellowish, slightly opalescent and free from visible particles. Do not administer solution that is discolored or contains a precipitate. Administer within 4 hr of reconstitution. Do not refrigerate or freeze reconstituted solution. Withdraw solution into syringe and

attach syringe to IV administration set. If multiple vials are used, vial contents may be pooled using a separate Mix2Vial transfer set for each vial. *Rate:* Infuse at a rate not to exceed 4 mL/min.

- **Y-Site Incompatibility:** Administer through separate infusion line. Do not mix with other medications or solutions.

Patient/Family Teaching

- Instruct patient to read the Patient Product Information before using and with each refill; new information may be available.
- Inform patient of signs and symptoms of hypersensitivity reactions; caution patient to notify health care professional promptly if these occur.
- Instruct patient to report bleeding to health care professional as a sign of immunogenicity.
- Advise patient to notify health care professional immediately if signs and symptoms of thrombosis (limb or abdomen swelling and/or pain, shortness of breath, loss of sensation or motor power, altered consciousness, vision, or speech) occur.
- Inform patient that because factor XIII concentrate is made from human blood, it may carry risk of transmitting infectious agents (viruses, Creutzfeldt-Jakob).
- Instruct patient to notify health care professional of all Rx or OTC medications, vitamins, or herbal products being taken and to avoid concurrent use of Rx, OTC, and herbal products, especially NSAIDs or aspirin without consulting health care professional.
- Advise patient to notify health care professional if planning to travel.
- Advise female patients to notify health care professional if pregnancy is planned or suspected or if breastfeeding.

Evaluation/Desired Outcomes

- Prevention of bleeding by replacement of deficient Factor XIII.

fentanyl (sublingual)
(**fen**-ta-nil)
Abstral

Classification
Thera: opioid analgesics
Pharm: opioid agonists

Schedule II

Pregnancy Category C

Indications
Management of breakthrough pain in opioid-tolerant cancer patients ≥18 yr who already receive opioids for persistent cancer-related pain (60 mg/day of oral morphine or equivalent).

Action
Binds to opiate receptors in the CNS, altering the response to and the perception of pain. **Therapeutic Effects:** ↓ breakthrough pain during chronic opioid therapy.

Pharmacokinetics
Absorption: 54% absorbed from oral mucosa following sublingual administration.
Distribution: Readily crosses the placenta and enters breast milk.
Metabolism and Excretion: >90% metabolized by the liver and intestinal mucosa (CYP3A4 enzyme system); <7% excreted unchanged in urine.
Half-life: *100 mcg*—5 hr, *200 mcg*—6.7 hr, *400 mcg*—13.5 hr, *800 mcg*—10 hr.

TIME/ACTION PROFILE

ROUTE	ONSET	PEAK	DURATION
SL	within 30 min	30–60 min	2–4 hr

Contraindications/Precautions
Contraindicated in: Opioid non-tolerant patients; Treatment of acute/post-operative pain including headache/migraine, dental pain or emergency room use; Lactation:

May cause sedation and/or respiratory depression.
Use Cautiously in: Geri: May be more sensitive to drug effects; Hepatic/renal impairment; OB: Use in pregnancy only if maternal benefit outweighs potential risk to fetus; chronic use may result in neonatal abstinence syndrome; Pedi: Safe and effective use in children <18 yr has not been established.
Exercise Extreme Caution in: Patients at risk for intracranial effects of CO_2 retention, including head injuries/ ↑ intracranial pressure.

Adverse Reactions/Side Effects
Opioid side effects ↑ with ↑ dosage. **CNS:** drowsiness, fatigue, headache, malaise, mood changes, weakness. **EENT:** blurred vision. **Resp:** RESPIRATORY DEPRESSION. **CV:** bradycardia, hypotension, tachycardia. **GI:** constipation, anorexia, nausea, abdominal pain, dry mouth, vomiting. **Derm:** rash, sweating. **Misc:** allergic reaction including ANAPHYLAXIS, physical dependence, psychological dependence.

Interactions
Drug-Drug: Should not be used within 14 days of **MAO inhibitors** because of possible severe and unpredictable reactions. **CNS depressants**, including other **opioids, sedative/ hypnotics, general anesthetics, phenothiazines, skeletal muscle relaxants, sedating antihistamines**, and **alcohol** may ↑ CNS depression, hypoventilation and hypotension. Concurrent use with **CYP3A4 inhibitors** including **ritonavir, ketoconazole, itraconazole, clarithromycin, nelfinavir, nefazodone, diltiazem, erythromycin, aprepitant, fluconazole, fosamprenavir**, and **verapamil** may significantly ↑ blood levels and ↑ risk of respiratory and CNS depression; careful monitoring and dose adjustment is recommended. Concurrent use of agents that induce **CYP3A4 enzyme** activity may ↓ analgesia. Administration of **partial-antagonistopioid analgesics** or **opioid**

antagonists will precipitate withdrawal in physically dependent patients.

Drug-Food: Grapefruit juice is a moderate inhibitor of the CYP3A4 enzyme system; concurrent use may ↑ blood levels and the risk of respiratory and CNS depression. Careful monitoring and dose adjustment is recommended.

Route/Dosage
SL (Adults): 100 mcg initially, then titrate using 100 mcg increments to provide adequate analgesia without undue side effects (not to exceed 2 doses per episode; no more than four doses per day; separate by at least 2 hrs).

Availability
Sublingual tablets: 100 mcg, 200 mcg, 300 mcg, 400 mcg, 600 mcg, 800 mcg.

NURSING IMPLICATIONS
Assessment
- Monitor type, location, and intensity of pain before and 1 hr after administration of sublingual fentanyl.
- Assess blood pressure, pulse, and respirations before and periodically during administration. If respiratory rate is <10 min, assess level of sedation. Physical stimulation may be sufficient to prevent hypoventilation. Subsequent doses may need to be ↓. Patients tolerant to opioid analgesics are usually tolerant to the respiratory depressant effects also.
- Monitor for application site reactions (paresthesia, ulceration, bleeding, pain, ulcer, irritation). Reactions are usually self-limited and rarely require discontinuation.
- *Lab Test Considerations:* May cause anemia, neutropenia, thrombocytopenia, and leukopenia.
- May cause hypokalemia, hypoalbuminemia, hypercalcemia, hypomagnesemia, and hyponatremia.
- *Toxicity and Overdose:* If an opioid antagonist is required to reverse respiratory depression or coma, naloxone (Narcan) is the antidote. Dilute the 0.4-mg ampule of naloxone in 10 mL of 0.9% NaCl and administer 0.5 mL (0.02 mg) by direct IV push every 2 min. For patients weighing <40 kg, dilute 0.1 mg of naloxone in 10 mL of 0.9% NaCl for a concentration of 10 mcg/mL and administer 0.5 mcg every 2 min. Use extreme caution when titrating dose in patients physically dependent on opioid analgesics to avoid withdrawal, seizures, and severe pain. Duration of respiratory depression may be longer than duration of opioid antagonist, requiring repeated doses.

Potential Nursing Diagnoses
Acute pain (Indications)
Risk for injury (Adverse Reactions)

Implementation
- *High Alert:* Accidental overdose of opioid analgesics has resulted in fatalities. Before administering, clarify all ambiguous orders; have second practitioner independently check original order and dose calculations.
- Patients considered opioid-tolerant are those who are taking ≥60 mg of oral morphine/day, at least 25 mcg transdermal fentanyl/hr, 30 mg of oxycodone/day, 8 mg of hydromorphone/day or an equianalgesic dose of another opioid for ≥1 wk.
- *High Alert:* Dose may be lethal to a child or individual not opioid tolerant; keep out of reach of children.
- Do not substitute fentanyl sublingual (Abstral) for fentanyl buccal (Fentora), fentanyl buccal soluble film (Onsolis), or fentanyl oral transmucosal (Actiq); doses are not equivalent.
- Available only through ABSTRAL REMS, a restricted distribution program. Only prescribers, pharmacies and distributors registered in the program and patients enrolled in the program have access. Program provides education, training, and counseling, regarding safe use of the medication. To enroll in the ABSTRAL REMS program call 1-888-227-8725 or visit www.abstralrems.com.
- Dose must start with 100 mcg initially, titrate to adequate pain relief, if initial dose is adequate, this will be the dose for subsequent breakthrough pain, if dose is inadequate within 30 min give

supplemental 100 mcg dose and ↑ next breakthrough dose by 100 mcg, if inadequate continue to ↑ breakthrough dose to 300, then 400, then 600 mcg then 800 mcg; limit treatment to 4 episodes/24 hr.

- If inadequate analgesia, a second dose may be used after 30 min. No more than 2 doses may be used to treat an episode of breakthrough pain. Episodes should be separated by at least 2 hrs. Other rescue medications may be used as directed.
- Once a successful dose has been established, if more than 4 breakthrough pain episodes/day occur, reevaluate opioid dose for persistent pain.
- **SL:** Place on the floor of the mouth directly under the tongue and allow to dissolve completely; do not chew, suck, or swallow. Do not eat or drink anything until tablet is dissolved. In patients with dry mouth, water may be used to moisten oral mucosa *before* taking sublingual fentanyl.

Patient/Family Teaching

- Instruct patient to take fentanyl sublingual tablets exactly as directed and to continue taking the around-the clock opioid pain medicine. Do not take more often than prescribed, keep out of reach of children, protect it from being stolen, and do not share with others, even if they have the same symptoms. Explain that fentanyl sublingual tablets may be fatal to children and individuals not tolerant to opioids. Advise patient to *Medication Guide* review each time Rx is refilled; new information may be available. Advise patient to notify health care professional if breakthrough pain is not alleviated or worsens.
- Explain ABSTRAL REMS Program to patient and caregiver. Patients must sign the Patient-Prescriber Agreement Form to confirm they understand the risks, appropriate use, and storage of fentanyl sublingual.
- Advise patient to dispose of unused fentanyl sublingual tablets by removing

from blister pack and flushing down toilet.

- Caution patient to make position changes slowly to minimize orthostatic hypotension.
- Medication causes dizziness and drowsiness. Advise patient to call for assistance during ambulation and transfer, and to avoid driving or other activities requiring alertness until response to medication is known.
- Instruct patient to avoid concurrent use of alcohol or other CNS depressants, such as sleep aids.
- Instruct patient to notify health care professional of all Rx or OTC medications, vitamins, or herbal products being taken and to avoid concurrent use of Rx, OTC, and herbal products without consulting health care professional.
- Advise patient to notify health care professional if pregnancy is planned or suspected or if breastfeeding.

Evaluation/Desired Outcomes

- ↓ in severity of pain during episodes of breakthrough pain in patients receiving long-acting opioids.

fingolimod
(fin-**go**-li-mod)
Gilenyna

Classification
Thera: anti-multiple sclerosis agents
Pharm: receptor modulators

Pregnancy Category C

Indications
Treatment of relapsing forms of multiple sclerosis.

Action
Converted by sphingosine kinase to the active metabolite fingolimod-phosphate, which binds to sphingosine 1-phosphate receptors, resulting in ↓ migration of lymphocytes into peripheral blood. This

may ↓ lymphocyte migration into the CNS. **Therapeutic Effects:** ↓ frequency of relapses/delayed accumulation of disability.

Pharmacokinetics

Absorption: Well absorbed (93%) following oral administration.

Distribution: Extensively distributed to body tissues; 86% of parent drug distributes into red blood cells; active metabolite uptake 17%.

Metabolism and Excretion: Converted to its active metabolite, then metabolized mostly by the CYP450 4F2 enzyme system, with further degradation by other enzyme systems. Most inactive metabolites excreted in urine (81%); <2.5% excreted as fingolimod and fingolimod-phosphate in feces.

Protein Binding: >99.7%.
Half-life: 6−9 hr.

TIME/ACTION PROFILE

ROUTE	ONSET	PEAK	DURATION
PO	unknown	1−2 mos*	2 mos†

*Time to steady state blood levels, peak blood levels after a single dose at 12−16 hr.
†Time for complete elimination.

Contraindications/Precautions

Contraindicated in: Active acute/chronic untreated infections; OB: Pregnancy; may cause fetal harm; Lactation: Breastfeeding should be avoided.

Use Cautiously in: Concurrent Class Ia or Class III antiarrhythmics, beta blockers, calcium channel blockers, bradycardia, history of syncope, ischemic heart disease or congestive heart failure (↑ risk of bradycardia/heart block); Severe hepatic impairment (↑ blood levels and risk of adverse reactions); Diabetes mellitus/history of uveitis (↑ risk of macular edema); Negative history for chickenpox or vaccination against varicella zoster virus vaccination; Geri: Use cautiously in patients >65 yr; risk of adverse reactions may be ↑ , consider age-related ↓ in cardiac/renal/hepatic function, chronic illnesses and concurrent drug therapy; Pedi: Safety and effectiveness not established for patients <18 yr.

Adverse Reactions/Side Effects

CNS: headache. **EENT:** blurred vision, eye pain, macular edema. **Resp:** cough, ↓ pulmonary function. **CV:** BRADYCARDIA, HEART BLOCK. **GI:** diarrhea, ↑ hepatic transaminases. **Hemat:** leukopenia, lymphopenia. **MS:** back pain. **Misc:** ↑ risk of infection.

Interactions

Drug-Drug: Concurrent use of **Class Ia or Class III antiarrhythmics** ↑ risk of serious arrhythmias; careful monitoring recommended. Concurrent use of **beta blockers** or **diltiazem** ↑ risk of bradycardia; careful monitoring recommended. Concurrent use of **ketoconazole** ↑ blood levels and of adverse reactions. ↑ risk of immunosuppression with **antineoplastics**, **immunosuppressants** or **immune modulating therapies**. **Live attenuated vaccines** ↑ risk of infection.

Route/Dosage

PO (Adults): 0.5 mg once daily.

Availability

Hard capsules: 0.5 mg.

NURSING IMPLICATIONS

Assessment

- Monitor for bradycardia for at least 6 hrs following first dose. Obtain baseline ECG before first dose if not recently available in patients at high risk for bradycardia. May cause AV conduction delays; usually transient and asymptomatic, resolving within first 24 hrs of therapy. May require treatment with atropine or isoproterenol. If fingolimod is discontinued for >2 wks, effects on heart rate and AV conduction may recur; use same precautions as for initial dosing.
- Monitor for signs of infection (fever, sore throat) during and for 2 mo after discontinuation of therapy. Consider suspending therapy if serious infection develops.
- Perform an opthalmologic exam prior to starting fingolimod, at 3−4 mo after treatment initiation, and if visual disturbances occur. Monitor visual acuity at baseline and during routine exams. Pa-

tients with diabetes or history of uveitis are at ↑ risk and should have regular ophthalmologic exams.

- Monitor pulmonary function tests for decline periodically during therapy. Obtain spirometry and diffusion lung capacity for carbon monoxide when indicated clincally.
- *Lab Test Considerations:* Obtain baseline liver function test before starting therapy. May cause ↑ liver transaminases. Monitor liver function tests if symptoms develop.
- Before initiating therapy, obtain a recent (within 6 mo) CBC. May cause ↓ lymphocyte counts.

Potential Nursing Diagnoses
Deficient knowledge, related to medication regimen (Patient/Family Teaching)

Implementation
- **PO:** Administer once daily without regard to food.

Patient/Family Teaching
- Instruct patient to take fingolimod as directed. Do not discontinue therapy without consulting health care professional. Advise patient to read the *Medication Guide* prior to starting therapy and with each Rx refill in case of changes.
- Advise patient to notify health care professional if signs and symptoms of liver dysfunction (unexplained nausea, vomiting, abdominal pain, fatigue, anorexia, jaundice, dark urine), infection, new onset of dyspnea, or changes in vision develop.
- Instruct patient not to receive live attenuated vaccines during and for 2 mo after treatment due to risk of infection. Patients who have not had chickenpox or vaccination should consider varicella zoster virus vaccination prior to starting therapy, then postponing start of fingolimod for 1 mo to allow for full effect of vaccination.
- Advise female patients to use contraception during and for at least 2 mo after discontinuation of therapy and to notify health care professional immediately if

pregnancy is planned or suspected or if breastfeeding. Encourage pregnant patients to enroll in the pregnancy registry by calling 1-877-598-7237.

Evaluation/Desired Outcomes
- Reduction in frequency of clinical exacerbations and delay of accumulation of physical disability in patients with relapsing forms of multiple sclerosis.

---

fosaprepitant (injection)
(fos-a-**prep**-i-tant)
Emend

Classification
Thera: antiemetics
Pharm: neurokinin antagonists

Pregnancy Category B

Indications
Prevention of nausea and vomiting associated with emetogenic chemotherapy.

Action
Acts as a selective antagonist at substance P/neurokinin₁ (NK1) receptors in the brain. **Therapeutic Effects:** ↓ nausea and vomiting associated with chemotherapy.

Pharmacokinetics
Absorption: Following IV administration, fosaprepitant is rapidly converted to aprepitant, the active component.
Distribution: Crosses the blood brain barrier; remainder of distribution unknown.
Metabolism and Excretion: Mostly metabolized by the liver (CYP3A4 enzyme system); not renally excreted.
Half-life: *Aprepitant*—9–13 hr.

TIME/ACTION PROFILE (antiemetic effect)

ROUTE	ONSET	PEAK	DURATION
PO	rapid	end of infusion*	24 hr

* Blood level.

Contraindications/Precautions

Contraindicated in: Hypersensitivity; Concurrent use with pimozide (risk of life-threatening adverse cardiovascular reactions); Lactation: May cause unwanted effects in nursing infants.

Use Cautiously in: OB: Use only if clearly needed; Pedi: Safety not established.

Adverse Reactions/Side Effects

CNS: dizziness, fatigue, weakness. **GI:** diarrhea. **Misc:** hiccups.

Interactions

Drug-Drug: Aprepitant inhibits, induces, and is metabolized by the CYP3A4 enzyme system; it also induces the CYP2C9 system. Concurrent use with other medications that are metabolized by CYP3A4 may result in ↑ toxicity from these agents including **docetaxel, paclitaxel, etoposide, irinotecan, ifosfamide, imatinib, vinorelbine, vinblastine, vincristine, midazolam, triazolam,** and **alprazolam**; concurrent use should be undertaken with caution. Concurrent use with drugs that significantly inhibit the CYP3A4 enzyme system including **ketoconazole, itraconazole, nefazodone, clarithromycin, ritonavir, nelfinavir,** and **diltiazem** may ↑ blood levels and effects of aprepitant. Concurrent use with drugs that induce the CYP3A4 enzyme system including **rifampin, carbamazepine,** and **phenytoin** may ↓ blood levels and effects of aprepitant. ↑ blood levels and effects of **dexamethasone**, (regimen reflects a 50% dose reduction); a similar effect occurs with **methylprednisolone** (IV dose by 25%, PO dose by 50% when used concurrently). May ↓ the effects of **warfarin** (careful monitoring for 2 wk recommended), **oral contraceptives** (use alternate method), **tolbutamide** and **phenytoin**.

Route/Dosage

IV (Adults): 115 mg 30 min prior to chemotherapy on day 1.

Availability

Lyophilized solid (requires reconstitution prior to injection): 115 mg/10-mL vial.

NURSING IMPLICATIONS

Assessment

- Assess nausea, vomiting, appetite, bowel sounds, and abdominal pain prior to and following administration.
- Monitor hydration, nutritional status, and intake and output. Patients with severe nausea and vomiting may require IV fluids in addition to antiemetics.
- *Lab Test Considerations:* Monitor clotting status closely during the 2–wk period, especially at 7–10 days, following fosaprepitant therapy in patients on chronic warfarin therapy.
- May cause mild, transient ↑ in alkaline phosphatase, AST, ALT, and BUN.
- May cause proteinuria, erythrocyturia, leukocyturia, hyperglycemia, hyponatremia, and ↑ leukocytes.
- May cause ↓ hemoglobin and WBC.

Potential Nursing Diagnoses

Risk for deficient fluid volume (Indications)

Imbalanced nutrition: less than body requirements (Indications)

Implementation

- Fosaprepitant is given as part of a regimen that includes a corticosteroid and a 5-HT$_3$ antagonist. Administer dexamethasone 12 mg PO and ondansetron 32 mg IV 30 min prior to chemotherapy treatment on day 1 of 3-day regimen.
- **Intermittent Infusion:** Inject 5 mL of 0.9% NaCl for Injection into vial. Swirl gently; avoid shaking or jetting saline into vial. *Diluent:* Prepare an infusion bag of 110 mL 0.9% NaCl. Withdraw entire volume from vial, and transfer to infusion bag for a total volume of 115 mL. *Concentration:* 1 mg/mL Gently invert bag 2–3 times. Solution is stable for 24 hr at room temperature. Inspect solution for particulate matter. Do not administer solutions that are discolored or contain particulate matter. *Rate:* Administer over 15 min.
- **Solution Incompatibility:** Incompatible with solutions containing divalent cations (calcium, magnesium) including LR and Hartmann's solution.

Patient/Family Teaching

- Instruct patient to notify health care professional if nausea and vomiting occur prior to administration.
- Advise patient to notify health care professional prior to taking any other Rx, OTC, or herbal products.
- Caution patient that fosaprepitant may ↓ the effectiveness of oral contraceptives. Advise patient to use alternate nonhormonal methods of contraception during and for 1 mo following treatment.
- Advise patient to notify health care professional if pregnancy is planned or suspected or if breastfeeding.
- Advise patient and family to use general measures to ↓ nausea (begin with sips of liquids and small, nongreasy meals; provide oral hygiene; remove noxious stimuli from environment).

Evaluation/Desired Outcomes

- ↓ nausea and vomiting associated with chemotherapy.

fospropofol
(foss-**pro**-po-fol)
Lusedra

Classification
Thera: general anesthetics

Pregnancy Category B

Indications

Monitored anesthesia care (MAC) in adults undergoing diagnositic/therapeutic procedures.

Action

Mechanism of action is not known. **Therapeutic Effects:** Induction and maintenance of anesthesia.

Pharmacokinetics

Absorption: Fospropofol is a prodrug that is rapidly converted by enzymatic action to propofol, the active drug. IV administration results in rapid conversion.
Distribution: Propofol crosses the placenta and breast milk.

Protein Binding: 98%.
Metabolism and Excretion: Propofol is highly metabolized, neglagible renal excretion.
Half-life: *Fospropofol*—0.9 hr; *Propofol from fospropofol*—1.1 hr.

TIME/ACTION PROFILE

ROUTE	ONSET	PEAK*	DURATION
IV	rapid	8 min	5 min

*Peak effect meaning time to sedation and duration measuring time to fully alert.

Contraindications/Precautions

Contraindicated in: None noted.
Use Cautiously in: Compromised cardiac function, reduced vascular tone or reduced intravascular volume (↑ risk of hypotension); Hepatic impairment; Renal impairment (safety not established for CCr <30 mL/min); Geri: Patients ≥65 yr or those with severe systemic disease (dose reduction required); OB, Lactation: Not recommended for use during labor, delivery or lactation (may cause neonatal respiratory and cardiovascular depression); Pedi: Children <18 yr (safety not established, use not recommended).

Adverse Reactions/Side Effects

Resp: RESPIRATORY DEPRESSION, cough, hypoxemia. **CV:** hypotension. **Derm:** pruritus. **Neuro:** paresthesia. **Misc:** loss of purposeful responsiveness.

Interactions

Drug-Drug: May ↑ risk of cardio-respiratory depression when used with other **cardio-respiratory depressants** including **benzodiazepines** and **opioid analgesics**.

Route/Dosage

Patients weighing >90 k g should be dosed as if they are 90 kg; patients weighing <60 kg should be dosed as if they are 60 kg.
IV (Adults): 6.5 mg/kg (not to exceed 16.5 mL) initially, followed by supplemental doses of 1.6 mg/kg (not to exceed 4 mL or more frequently that every 4 min) as needed.

Route/Dosage
IV (Geriatric Patients ≥65 yr or those with severe systemic disease): 75% of standard dose.

Availability
Solution for injection: 1050 mg/30 mL.

NURSING IMPLICATIONS

Assessment
- Assess respiratory status, pulse, and blood pressure continuously throughout fospropofol therapy. May cause apnea. Use supplemental O₂ for all patients receiving fospropofol. Fospropofol should be used only by individuals experienced in endotracheal intubation, and equipment for this procedure should be readily available.
- Assess level of sedation and level of consciousness throughout and following administration.
- *Toxicity and Overdose:* If overdose occurs, monitor pulse, respiration, and blood pressure continuously. Maintain patent airway and assist ventilation as needed. If hypotension occurs, treatment includes IV fluids, repositioning, and vasopressors.

Potential Nursing Diagnoses
Ineffective breathing pattern (Adverse Reactions)
Risk for injury (Side Effects)

Implementation
- Dose is titrated to patient response. Administer supplemental doses based on level of sedation and level of sedation required for procedure; only when patient demonstrates purposeful movement in response to verbal or light tactile stimulation and no more frequently than every 4 min.
- Fospropofol has no effect on the pain threshold. Adequate analgesia should *always* be used when fospropofol is used as an adjunct to surgical procedures.

IV Administration
- **Direct IV:** *Diluent:* Administer undiluted. Shake well before use. Solution is clear and colorless; do not administer

solutions that are discolored or contain a precipitate. Contains no preservatives; maintain sterile technique and administer immediately after preparation. *Concentration:* Undiluted: 35mg/mL.
- Discard unused portions and IV lines at the end of anesthetic procedure. *Rate:* Administer over 3−5 min through a free-flowing IV line. Titrate to desired level of sedation. Flush line with 0.9% NaCl before and after administration.
- **Solution Compatibility:** D5W, 0.9% NaCl, 0.45% NaCl, LR, D5/LR, D5/0.45% NaCl, D5/0.2% NaCl, D5/0.45% NaCl with 20 mEq KClDo not mix with other drugs or fluids prior to administration.
- **Y-Site Incompatibility:** meperidine, midazolam.

Patient/Family Teaching
- Inform patient that this medication will ↓ mental recall of the procedure.
- Inform patient that paresthesias (burning, tingling, stinging) and pruritus in the perineal region may occur upon injection of fospropofol; usually mild to moderate intensity, last a short time, and require no treatment.
- May cause drowsiness or dizziness. Advise patient to request assistance prior to ambulation and transfer and to avoid driving or other activities requiring alertness for 24 hr following administration.
- Advise patient to avoid alcohol or other CNS depressants without the advice of a health care professional for 24 hr following administration.

Evaluation/Desired Outcomes
- Induction and maintenance of anesthesia.
- Amnesia.
- Sedation in mechanically ventilated patients in an intensive care setting.

---

glycopyrrolate oral solution
(glye-koe-**pye**-roe-late)
Cuvposa

Indications

Prevention of excessive drooling associated with neurologic conditions in patients 3-16 yr.

Action

Competitively inhibits peripheral cholinergic receptors, including salivary glands. **Therapeutic Effects:** ↓ problem drooling.

Pharmacokinetics

Absorption: Absorption following oral administration is low and variable; absorption is ↓ by a high fat meal.
Distribution: Unknown.
Metabolism and Excretion: Excreted mostly unchanged in urine (65–80%), small amount eliminated as metabolites.
Half-life: 3–3.2 hr.

TIME/ACTION PROFILE

ROUTE	ONSET	PEAK†	DURATION
PO	unknown	2.6–3.1 hr	6–8 hr

†Blood levels.

Contraindications/Precautions

Contraindicated in: Conditions or concurrent drug therapy for which anticholinergic therapy is contraindicated including glaucoma, paralytic ileus, unstable cardiovascular status due to acute hemorrhage, severe ulcerative colitis, toxic megacolon as a complication of ulcerative colitis, myasthenia gravis; Concurrent use of potassium chloride capsules or tablets (passage through GI tract may be delayed).
Use Cautiously in: High ambient temperatures; ↑ risk of heat prostration (fever and heat stroke) due to ↓ sweating); Renal impairment; Autonomic neuropathy; Ulcerative colitis (↑ doses may ↑ risk of paralytic ileus ["toxic megacolon"]); Hyperthyroidism; Coronary heart disease, congestive heart failure, cardiac tachyarrhythmias, tachycardia, or hypertension; Hiatal hernia (may aggravate reflux esophagitis); OB: Use in pregnant women only if clearly needed; Lactation: Use cautiously during lactation; Pedi: Safety and effectiveness not established in children <3 yr.

Adverse Reactions/Side Effects

CNS: SEIZURES, headache, abnormal behavior, agression, agitation, crying, drowsiness, irritability, moaning, mood alteration, poor impulse control, restlessness. **EENT:** nasal congestion, blurred vision, nasal dryness, nystagmus. **Resp:** ↑ viscosity of secretions. **CV:** tachycardia. **GI:** INCOMPLETE MECHANICAL INTESTINAL OBSTRUCTION, constipation, dry mouth, vomiting, abdominal discomfort, abdominal distention, abnormal taste, chapped lips, diarrhea, flatulence, intestinal pseudo-obstruction. **GU:** urinary retention. **Derm:** flushing, dry skin, pallor, pruritus, rash. **F and E:** dehydration.

Interactions

Drug-Drug: May ↑ levels of **digoxin**, **atenolol**, or **metformin** levels; consider dose reductions or other changes in therapy. Effects may be ↑ by **amantadine**; consider ↓ dose of glycoypyrrolate. May ↓ levels of **haloperidol** or **levodopa**; ↑ glycoypyrrolate dose may be required.

Route/Dosage

PO (Children 3–16 yr): 0.02 mg/kg three times daily initially; titrate in increments of 0.02 mg/kg every 5-7 days (not to exceed 0.1 mg/kg three times daily or 1.5-3 mg per dose).

Availability

Oral solution (cherry): 1 mg/5 mL.

NURSING IMPLICATIONS

Assessment

● Assess for constipation (abdominal distension, pain, nausea, vomiting), especially within 4–5 days of initial dose or after dose ↑ .

Potential Nursing Diagnoses

Risk for constipation (Adverse Reactions)
Risk for imbalanced body temperature
(Adverse Reactions)

Implementation

- **PO:** Administer at least 1 hr before or 2 hrs after meals.

Patient/Family Teaching

- Instruct patient or parent to take glycopyrrolate as directed. Use an accurate measuring device (dosing cup) for correct dosing and administer with an oral syringe to ensure dose is taken. Dosing is started low and titrated slowly over several wk; do not ↑ dose without consulting health care professional. Advise patient/parent to read *Patient and Caregiver Information* prior to starting therapy and with each Rx refill.
- May cause drowsiness or blurred vision. Caution patient to avoid driving or other activities requiring alertness until response to medication is known.
- If constipation, diarrhea, signs of urinary retention (inability to urinate, dry diapers or undergarments, irritability, crying), or signs of hypersensitivity (rash, hives, allergic reaction) occur, stop administering glycopyrrolate and notify health care professional.
- May cause ↓ sweating; avoid overheating. Avoid exposure to hot or very warm environments and notify health care professional immediately if signs of heatstroke (hot, red skin; ↓ alertness or unconsciousness, fast, weak pulse; fast, shallow breathing; ↑ temperature.
- Advise patient to notify health care professional if pregnancy is planned or suspected or if breastfeeding.

Evaluation/Desired Outcomes

- ↓ in chronic, severe drooling.

---

hydroxyprogesterone caproate

(hye-drox-ee-pro-**jess**-te-rone **kap**-roe-ate)
Makena

Classification
Thera: hormones
Pharm: progestins

Pregnancy Category B

Indications

To ↓ the risk of preterm birth in women with a singleton pregnancy who have a history of previous singleton preterm birth.

Action

A synthetic analog of progesterone. Produces secretory changes in the endometrium. ↑ s basal temperature. Produces changes in the vaginal epithelium. Relaxes uterine smooth muscle. Stimulates mammary alveolar growth. Inhibits pituitary function. Action in reducing risk of recurrent preterm birth is unknown. **Therapeutic Effects:** ↓ risk of preterm birth in women at risk.

Pharmacokinetics

Absorption: Slowly absorbed following IM administration.
Distribution: Unknown.
Protein Binding: Extensively bound to plasma proteins.
Metabolism and Excretion: Extensively metabolized by the liver.
Half-life: 7.8 days.

TIME/ACTION PROFILE (blood levels)

ROUTE	ONSET	PEAK	DURATION
IM	unknown	4.6 days	7 days

Contraindications/Precautions

Contraindicated in: Hypersensitivity to hydroxyprogesterone or castor oil; History of or known thrombosis/thromboembolic disorder; History of or known/suspected breast cancer or other hormone-sensitive cancer; Unexplained abnormal vaginal bleeding unrelated to pregnancy; Cholestatic jaundice of pregnancy; Benign/malignant liver tumors or active liver disease; Uncontrolled hypertension.
Use Cautiously in: Risk factors for thromboembolic disorders (may ↑ risk); Diabetes mellitus or risk factors for

diabetes mellitus (may impair glucose tolerance); History of preeclampsia, epilepsy, cardiac or renal impairment (may be adversely affected by fluid retention); History of depression (may worsen); Safe and effective use in children <16 yr has not been established.

Adverse Reactions/Side Effects
CNS: depression. **CV:** hypertension. **GI:** diarrhea, jaundice, nausea. **Derm:** <u>urticaria, pruritus.</u> **F and E:** fluid retention. **Hemat:** THROMBOEMBOLISM. **Local:** <u>injections site reactions.</u> **Misc:** allergic reactions including ANGIOEDEMA.

Interactions
Drug-Drug: May ↑ metabolism and ↓ blood levels and effectiveness of **drugs metabolized by the CYP1A2, CYP2A6 and CYP2B6 enzyme systems**.

Route/Dosage
IM (Adults): 250 mg once weekly starting between 16 wks, 0 days and 20 wks, 6 days continuing until wk 37 of gestation or delivery, whichever occurs first.

Availability
Solution for IM injection (contains castor oil): 1250 mg/5 mL vial (250 mg/mL).

NURSING IMPLICATIONS

Assessment
- Monitor for signs and symptoms of thromboembolic disorders throughout therapy.
- Monitor vital signs during therapy. If hypertension occurs, consider discontinuation of therapy.
- Assess for signs and symptoms of allergic reactions (urticaria, pruritus, angioedema) during therapy. Consider discontinuation if allergic reactions occur.
- Monitor for fluid retention during therapy, especially in patients at ↑ risk for complications (preeclampsia, epilepsy, migraine, asthma, cardiac or renal dysfunction).
- Assess mental status and mood changes, especially in women with a history of

depression. Discontinue hydroxyprogesterone if depression recurs or worsens.
- *__Lab Test Considerations:__* May ↓ glucose tolerance. Monitor serum glucose in prediabetic and diabetic women during therapy.

Potential Nursing Diagnoses
Deficient knowledge, related to disease process and medication regimen (Patient/Family Teaching)

Implementation
- **IM:** Draw up 1 mL of solution into a 3 mL syringe with an 18 gauge needle. Solution is clear, yellow, viscous and oily. Do not administer solutions that are cloudy or contain particles. Change needle to 21 gauge 1 1/2 inch needle. Inject into upper outer quadrant of gluteus maximus slowly, over 1 min or longer. Apply pressure to injection site to minimize bruising and swelling. Store hydroxyprogesterone in original box, at room temperature, protected from light. Discard unused product after 5 wks from first use.

Patient/Family Teaching
- Instruct patient to continue to receive injection weekly from health care professional. If a dose is missed, consult health care professional for instructions regarding returning to schedule.
- Advise patient to notify health care professional if signs and symptoms of blood clots (leg swelling, redness in your leg, a spot on your leg that is warm to touch, leg pain that worsens when you bend your foot), allergic reactions (hives, itching, swelling of the face), depression, or yellowing of skin and whites of the eyes occur.
- Inform patient that injection site reactions (pain, swelling, itching, bruising, nodule formation) may occur. If ↑ pain over time, oozing of blood or fluid, or swelling occur, notify health care professional.

Evaluation/Desired Outcomes

- ↓ risk of preterm birth in women at risk.

---

ipilimumab
(i-pil-**li**-moo-mab)
Yervoy

Classification
Thera: antineoplastics
Pharm: monoclonal antibodies

Pregnancy Category C

Indications

Treatment of unresectable/metastatic melanoma.

Action

Binds to cytotoxic T-lymphocyte-associated agntigen 4 (CTLA-4). CTLA-4 is a negative regulator of T-cell activation; binding results in augmented T-cell activation and proliferation. **Therapeutic Effects:** ↓ spread of melanoma.

Pharmacokinetics

Absorption: IV administration results in complete bioavailability.
Distribution: Crosses the placenta.
Metabolism and Excretion: Unknown.
Half-life: 14.7 days.

TIME/ACTION PROFILE

ROUTE	ONSET	PEAK	DURATION
IV	unknown	unknown	unknown

Contraindications/Precautions

Contraindicated in: Lactation: Avoid breastfeeding.
Use Cautiously in: OB: use only if potential maternal benefit justifies potential risk to the fetus; may cause fetal harm; Pedi: safe and effective use in children has not been established.

Adverse Reactions/Side Effects

CNS: fatigue. **EENT:** immune-mediated ocular disease. **GI:** IMMUNE-MEDIATED COLITIS, IMMUNE-MEDIATED HEPATITIS, colitis, diarrhea. **Derm:** immune-mediated dermatitis including TOXIC EPIDERMAL NECROLYSIS, pruritus, rash. **Endo:** IMMUNE-MEDIATED ENDOCRINOPATHIES including HYPOPITUITARISM, HYPOTHYROIDISM, HYPERTHRYRODISM, ADRENAL INSUFFICIENCY, CUSHING'S SYDROME, AND HYPOGONADISM. **Neuro:** IMMUNE-MEDIATED NEUROPATHY.

Interactions

Drug-Drug: None noted.

Route/Dosage

IV (Adults): 3 mg/kg every three wk for a total of four doses.

Availability

Solution for IV infusion (requires further dilution): 50 mg/10 mL vial, 200 mg/40 mL vial.

NURSING IMPLICATIONS

Assessment

- Monitor for signs and symptoms of entercolitis (diarrhea, abdominal pain, mucus or blood in stool, with or without fever) and bowel perforation (peritoneal signs, ileus). Rule out infection and consider endoscopic evaluation. If severe enterocolitis occurs, discontinue ilipimumab and start systemic corticosteroids at doses of 1–2 mg/kg/day of prednisone or equivalents. At improvement to Grade 1 or less, taper corticosteroid over at least 1 month. Withhold dose for moderate enterocolitis; administer anti-diarrheal treatment and if persists for >1 wk, start corticosteroids at a dose of 0.5 mg/kg/day of prednisone or equivalent.
- Assess for signs and symptoms of hepatotoxicity (yellowing of skin or whites of eyes, unusual darkening of urine, unusual tiredness, pain in right upper stomach) before each dose. If hepatotoxicity occurs, rule out infectious or malignant causes. Permanently discontinue ipilimumab if Grade 3–5 hepatotoxicity occurs and start systemic corticosteroids at a dose of 1–2 mg/kg/day of prednisone or equivalent. When liver function tests show sustained improvement or return to baseline, start corticosteroid taper over 1 month. May administer mycophenolate in patients with

persistent severe hepatitis despite high-dose corticosteroids. Withhold ipilimumab in patients with Grade 2 hepatotoxicity.

- Monitor for signs and symptoms of dermatitis (rash, pruritus). Unless other causes are identified, assume immune-mediated dermatitis. Permanently discontinue ipilimumab in patients with Stevens-Johnson syndrome, toxic epidermal necrolysis, or rash complicated by full thickness dermal ulceration, or necrotic, bullous, or hemorrhagic manifestations. Administer corticosteroids at a dose of 1 – 2 mg/kg/day of prednisone or equivalent. When dermatitis is controlled, taper corticosteroids over at least 1 month. Withhold ipilimumab in patients with moderate to severe signs and symptoms. Treat mild to moderate dermatitis symptomatically. Administer topical or systemic corticosteroids if there is no improvement of symptoms within 1 wk.

- Monitor for symptoms of motor or sensory neuropathy (unilateral or bilateral weakness, sensory alterations, paresthesia). Permanently discontinue ipilimumab in patients with severe neuropathy (interfering with daily activities). Institute treatment as needed. Consider systemic corticosteroids of 1 – 2 mg/kg/day of prednisone or equivalent for severe neuropathy. Withhold dose of ipilimumab in patients with moderate neuropathy (not interfering with daily activities).

- Monitor for clinical signs and symptoms of hypophysitis, adrenal insufficiency (including adrenal crisis), and hyper or hypothyroidism (fatigue, headache, mental status changes, abdominal pain, unusual bowel habits, hypotension) Unless other causes are determined, consider signs and symptoms as immune-mediated endocrinopathies. Withhold ipilimumab in symptomatic patients and initiate corticosteroids at 1 – 2 mg/kg/day of prednisone or equivalents. Initiate hormone replacement therapy as needed.

- Assess eyes for signs and symptoms of uveitis, iritis, or episcleritis. Administer corticosteroid eyedrops if these occur. Permanently discontinue ipilimumab for immune-mediated occular disease unresponsive to local immunosuppressive therapy.

- ***Lab Test Considerations:*** Monitor liver function tests (AST, ALT, bilirubin) periodically during therapy; ↑ frequency of monitoring if levels ↑ .

- Monitor thyroid function tests and serum chemistries at start of therapy, before each dose, and as clinically indicated.

Potential Nursing Diagnoses
Impaired skin integrity (Indications)

Implementation

- Withhold dose for any moderate immune-mediated adverse reactions or for symptomatic endocrinopathy. For patients with complete or partial resolution of adverse reactions (Grade 0 – 1), who are receiving equivalents of <7.5 mg prednisone/day, resume isilimumab at a dose of 3 mg/kg every 3 wks until administration of all 4 planned doses or 16 wks from 1st dose, whichever occurs earlier.

- Permanently discontinue if persistent moderate adverse reactions or inability to reduce corticosteroid dose to equivalent of prednisone 7.5 mg/day, failure to complete full treatment course within 16 wks from infusion of 1st dose, or severe or life threatening adverse reactions occur including: Colitis with abdominal pain, fever, or peritoneal signs; ↑ in stool frequency of 7 or more over baseline, stool incontinence. need for IV hydration for >24 hrs, GI hemorrhage and GI perforation; AST or ALT >5 times the upper limits of normal or total bilirubin >3 times the upper limit of normal; Stevens-Johnson syndome, toxic epidermal necrolysis, or rash complicated by full-thickness dermal ulceration, or necrotic, bullous, or hemorrhagic manifestations; Severe motor or sensory neuropathy, Guillian-

Barre syndrome, or myasthenia gravis; Severe immune-mediated reactions involving any organ system (nephritis, pneumonitis, pancreatitis, non-infectious myocarditis); and Immune-mediated ocular disease that is unresponsive to topical immunosuppressive therapy.

- Allow vial to stand at room temperature for 5 min prior to preparation of infusion. Withdraw amount of ipilimumab required and transfer to IV bag. *Diluent:* Dilute with 0.9% NaCL or D5W. *Concentration:* 1 mg/mL to 2 mg/mL Mix slowly by gentle inversion; do not shake. Solution is clear, pale yellow, and may contain translucent-to-white amorphous particles; do not administer if cloudy, discolored, or contains particulate matter. Store for up to 24 hr at room temperature or refrigerated; do not freeze, protect from light. Discard partially used vials. *Rate:* Infuse over 90 min through a sterile, non-pyrogenic, low-protein-binding in-line filter. Flush the IV line with 0.9% NaCl or D5W after each dose.
- **Y-Site Incompatibility:** Do not mix with or infuse with other solutions or products.

Patient/Family Teaching
- Inform patient of the risk of immune-mediated reactions due to T-cell activation and proliferation. Advise patients these may be severe and fatal. Instruct patient to notify health care professional immediately if signs and symptoms occur.
- Instruct patient to read the *Medication Guide* before starting therapy and before each dose of ipilimumab.
- Advise female patients to notify health care professional if pregnancy is planned or suspected or if breastfeeding. Contraception should be used throughout therapy. Women must choose to discontinue breastfeeding or ipilimumab.

Evaluation/Desired Outcomes
- ↓ spread of melanoma.

---

ivermectin
(eye-ver-**mek**-tin)
Stromectol

Classification
Thera: anthelmintics
Pharm: avermectins

Pregnancy Category C

Indications
Intestinal strongyloidiasis. Onchocerciasis (nemotode form only).

Action
Binds selectively and with a high affinity to chloride channels in invertebrate nerve and muscle cells, resulting in parasite paralysis and death. Active against *Strongyloides stercoralis* and the nemotode form of *Onchocerca volvulus*. **Therapeutic Effects:** Death of infecting parasites with resolution of symptoms of infection.

Pharmacokinetics
Absorption: Some absorption follows oral administration; fat enhances absorption.
Distribution: Small amounts enter breast milk.
Metabolism and Excretion: Metabolized by the liver; parent drug and metabolites excreted mainly in feces; <1% excreted unchanged in urine.
Half-life: 18 hr.

TIME/ACTION PROFILE (blood levels)

ROUTE	ONSET	PEAK	DURATION
PO	unknown	4 hr	unknown

Contraindications/Precautions
Contraindicated in: Hypersensitivity; OB: Safe use in pregnancy has not been established.
Use Cautiously in: Lactation: Use only if risk of delayed treatment outweighs possible risk to newborn; Pedi: Safe and effective use in children <15 kg has not been established.

Adverse Reactions/Side Effects
CNS: dizziness, drowsiness, fatigue, vertigo, weakness. **GI:** abdominal pain, ano-

rexia, constipation, diarrhea, nausea, vomiting. **Derm:** pruritus, rash, urticaria. **Neuro:** tremor. **Misc:** Mazzotti reaction (onchocerciasis only).

Interactions
Drug-Drug: May ↑ risk of bleeding with **warfarin**.

Route/Dosage
Strongyloidiasis
PO (Adults and Children): 200 mcg/kg as a single dose (≥*80 kg*— 200 mcg/kg, *66–79 kg*—5 tablets, *51–65 kg*—4 tablets, *36–50 kg*—3 tablets, *25–35 kg*—2 tablets, *15–24 kg*—1 tablet).

Onchocerciasis
PO (Adults and Children): 150 mcg/kg as a single dose (≥*85 kg*— 150 mcg/kg, *65–84 kg*—4 tablets, *45–64 kg*—3 tablets, *26–44 kg*—2 tablets, *15–25 kg*—1 tablet); course may be repeated at 3–12 mo intervals.

Availability
Tablets: 3 mg.

NURSING IMPLICATIONS

Assessment
- Monitor repeat stool samples for clearance of infection.
- Monitor for signs and symptoms of Mazzotti reactions (arthralgia/synovitis, enlargement and tenderness of axillary cervical, inguinal and other lymph nodes, skin involvement including edema, papular and pustular or frank urticarial rash, fever) in patients treated for Onchocerciasis. Treatment includes oral hydration, recumbency, IV normal saline, and/or parenteral corticosteroids to treat postural hypotension, and antihistamines and/or aspirin for most mild to moderate cases.
- *Lab Test Considerations:* May rarely cause ↑ INR when co-administered with warfarin.
- May cause ↑ ALT and ↑ AST.
- May cause ↓ leukocyte count, eosinophilia, and ↑ hemoglobin.

Potential Nursing Diagnoses
Risk for infection (Indications)

Implementation
- **PO:** Administer on an empty stomach with water.

Patient/Family Teaching
- Instruct patient to take the single dose on an empty stomach with water.
- Advise patient that ivermectin does not kill the adult Onchocerca parasites; repeated follow-up and retreatment is usually required.
- Advise female patient to notify health care professional if pregnancy is planned or suspected or if breastfeeding.

Evaluation/Desired Outcomes
- Eradication of Strongyloidiasis and Onchocerca infections.

Japanese encephalitis virus vaccine
(Ja-pan-**ees** en-se-fa-**li**-tes vak-**seen**)
Ixiaro

Classification
Thera: vaccines/immunizing agents

Pregnancy Category B

Indications
Active immunization against disease caused by Japanese encephalitis virus (JEV) in persons ≥17 yr.

Action
An inactive form of the virus induces antibodies that neutralize live JEV. **Therapeutic Effects:** Prevention of disease caused by JEV.

Pharmacokinetics
Absorption: Absorption follows intramuscular administration.
Distribution: Unknown.
Metabolism and Excretion: Unknown.

Half-life: Unknown.

TIME/ACTION PROFILE (antibody production)

ROUTE	ONSET	PEAK	DURATION
IM	unknown	within 10 days	unknown

Contraindications/Precautions

Contraindicated in: Serious hypersensitivity to a previous dose; Serious hypersensitivity to protamine.
Use Cautiously in: Immunocompromised patients (may have ↓ response); OB, Lactation: Safety and effectiveness not established; Pedi: Safety and effectiveness not established.

Adverse Reactions/Side Effects

CNS: headache. **Local:** pain, tenderness, edema, pruritus. **MS:** myalgia.

Interactions

Drug-Drug: Concurrent use of immunosuppressives including antineoplastics and corticosteroids may ↓ antibody reponse and ↑ risk of adverse reactions.

Route/Dosage

IM (Adults ≥17 yr): 0.5 mL, repeated 28 days later; series completed at least 1 wk prior to potential exposure to JEV.

Availability

Suspension for injection (contains protamine): 0.5 mL single dose syringes.

NURSING IMPLICATIONS

Assessment

- Determine if patient has had reactions to previous vaccines.
- Obtain temperature. Vaccine should not be administered to patients with fever >100°F.

Potential Nursing Diagnoses

Risk for infection (Indications)

Implementation

- Immunization is administered in 2 doses, 28 days apart, completed at least 1 wk prior to exposure to JEV.
- **IM:** Store in refrigerator; clear liquid with white precipitation may form during storage. Shake syringe well to obtain a white, opaque, homogenous suspen-

sion. Do not administer if discolored or contains particulate matter. Inject into deltoid; do not give intravenously, intradermally or subcutaneously.

Patient/Family Teaching

- Inform patient of the purpose of vaccine and that vaccine is non-infectious. If second dose is missed, contact health care professional to determine when to receive second dose. Maximum protection is not achieved until 1 wk after second dose. Advise patient to read *Patient Information Sheet* prior to vaccination.
- Advise patient of precautions to take to reduce exposure to mosquito bites transmitting virus (adequate clothing, use of repellents, mosquito nets). Vaccine may not fully protect everyone who gets the vaccine, does not protect against other types of encephalitis or other diseases transmitted by mosquito bites.
- Advise patient to tell health care professional what medications they are taking.
- Advise female patients to notify health care professional if pregnancy is planned or suspected, or if breastfeeding.

Evaluation/Desired Outcomes

- Protection against Japanese Encephalitis Virus.

---

lacosamide
(la-**kose**-a-mide)
Vimpat

Classification
Thera: anticonvulsants

Schedule V

Pregnancy Category C

Indications

Adjunctive therapy of partial-onset seizures.

Action

Mechanism is not known, but may involve enhancement of slow inactivation of sodium channels with resultant membrane stabilization; also binds to collapsin response mediator protein-2 (CRMP-2) which is involved in neural differentiation and growth. **Therapeutic Effects:** ↓ incidence and severity of partial-onset seizures.

Pharmacokinetics

Absorption: 100% absorbed following oral administration; IV administration results in complete bioavailability.

Distribution: Unknown.

Metabolism and Excretion: Partially metabolized by the liver; 40% excreted in urine as unchanged drug, 30% as a metabolite.

Half-life: 13 hr.

TIME/ACTION PROFILE (blood levels)

ROUTE	ONSET	PEAK	DURATION
PO	unknown	1–4 hr	12 hr
IV	unknown	end of infusion	12 hr

Contraindications/Precautions

Contraindicated in: Hypersensitivity; Severe hepatic impairment; Lactation: Lacatation.

Use Cautiously in: CCr <30 mL/min (use lower daily dose); All patients (may ↑ risk of suicidal thoughts/behaviors); Mild to moderate hepatic impairment; titrate dose carefully, use lower daily dose; Known cardiac conduction problems or severe cardiac disease (MI or CHF); OB: Use during pregnancy only if potential benefit justifies risk to the fetus; Pedi: Children <17 yr (safety and effectiveness not established); Geri: Titrate dose carefully.

Adverse Reactions/Side Effects

CNS: SUICIDAL THOUGHTS, dizziness, headache, syncope, vertigo. **EENT:** diplopia. **CV:** PR interval prolongation. **GI:** nausea, vomiting. **Neuro:** ataxia. **Misc:** physical dependence, psychological dependence, multiorgan hypersensitivity reactions (Drug Reaction with Eosinophilia and Systemic Symptoms—DRESS).

Interactions

Drug-Drug: Use cautiously with other **drugs that affect cardiac conduction**.

Route/Dosage

PO, IV (Adults): 50 mg twice daily; may be ↑ weekly by 100 mg/day in two divided doses up to a maintenance dose of 200–400 mg/day given in two divided doses.

Hepatic/Renal Impairment

PO, IV (Adults): *CCr ≤30 mL/min or mild to moderate hepatic impairment*— daily dose should not exceed 300 mg.

Availability

Tablets: 50 mg, 150 mg, 200 mg. **Solution for injection:** 10 mg/mL.

NURSING IMPLICATIONS

Assessment

- Assess location, duration, and characteristics of seizure activity. Institute seizure precautions.
- Monitor closely for notable changes in behavior that could indicate the emergence or worsening of suicidal thoughts or behavior or depression.
- Assess ECG prior to therapy in patients with pre-existing cardiac disease.
- *Lab Test Considerations:* May cause ↑ ALT, which may return to normal without treatment.

Potential Nursing Diagnoses

Risk for injury (Indications)

Implementation

- IV administration is indicated for short term replacement when PO administration is not feasible. When switching from PO to IV, initial total daily dose should be equivalent to total daily dose and frequency of PO therapy. At end of IV period, may switch to PO at equivalent daily dose and frequency of IV therapy.
- **PO:** May be administered with or without food.

- **Intermittent Infusion:** *Diluent:* May be administered undiluted or diluted with 0.9% NaCl, D5W, or LR. *Concentration:* 10 mg/mL Solution is clear and colorless; do not administer solutions that are discolored or contain a precipitate. Solution is stable for 24 hr at room temperature. Discard unused portion. *Rate:* Infuse over 30–60 min.

Patient/Family Teaching

- Instruct patient to take lacosamide around the clock, as directed. Medication should be gradually discontinued over at least 1 wk to prevent seizures. Advise patient to read the *Medication Guide* before starting therapy and with each Rx refill.
- May cause dizziness, ataxia, and syncope. Caution patient to avoid driving or other activities requiring alertness until response to medication is known. Tell patient not to resume driving until physician gives clearance based on control of seizure disorder. If syncope occurs, advise patient to lay down with legs raised until recovered and notify health care professional.
- Inform patients and families of risk of suicidal thoughts and behavior and advise that behavioral changes, emergency or worsening signs and symptoms of depression, unusual changes in mood, or emergence of suicidal thoughts, behavior, or thoughts of self-harm should be reported to health care professional immediately.
- Instruct patient to notify health care professional if signs of multiorgan hypersensitivity reactions (fever, rash, fatigue, jaundice, dark urine) occur.
- Advise patient to consult health care professional before taking other Rx, OTC, or herbal preparation and to avoid taking alcohol or other CNS depressants concurrently with lacosamide.
- Advise female patients to notify health care professional if pregnancy is planned or suspected or if breast feeding. Encourage pregnant patients to enroll in the pregnancy registry by calling 1-888-537-7734.

Evaluation/Desired Outcomes

- ↓ seizure activity.

liraglutide
(lir-a-**gloo**-tide)
Victoza

Classification
Thera: antidiabetics
Pharm: Glucagon-Like Peptide-1 (GLP-1) receptor agonists

Pregnancy Category C

Indications

Adjunct treatment to diet and exercise in the management of adults with type 2 diabetes mellitus; not recommended as first line therapy, a substitute for insulin, use in patients with type 1 diabetes or ketoacidosis.

Action

Acts as an acylated human Glucagon-Like Peptide-1 (GLP-1, an incretin) receptor agonist; ↑ s intracellular cyclic AMP (cAMP) leading to insulin release when glucose is elevated, which then subsides as blood glucose ↓ s toward euglycemia. Also ↓ s glucagon secretion and delays gastric emptying. **Therapeutic Effects:** Improved glycemic control.

Pharmacokinetics

Absorption: 55% absorbed following subcutaneous injection.
Distribution: Unknown.
Protein Binding: >98%.
Metabolism and Excretion: Endogenously metabolized.
Half-life: 13 hr.

TIME/ACTION PROFILE (↓ in HbA_{1c})

ROUTE	ONSET	PEAK	DURATION
Subcut	within 4 wk	8 wk	unknown

Contraindications/Precautions

Contraindicated in: Personal or family history of Medullary Thyroid Carcinoma (MTC)/Multiple Endocrine Neoplasia syndrome type 2 (MEN 2); Lactation: Avoid use during breastfeeding; Pedi: Not recommended in children.

Use Cautiously in: History of pancreatitis; Hepatic/renal impairment; OB: Use during pregnancy only if potential benefit justifies potential risk to fetus.

Adverse Reactions/Side Effects

CNS: headache. **GI:** diarrhea, nausea, vomiting, constipation, pancreatitis. **Local:** injection site reactions.

Interactions

Drug-Drug: Concurrent use with **agents that ↑ insulin secretion** including **sulfonylureas** may ↑ the risk of serious hypoglycemia, use cautiously and consider dose reduction of agent increasing insulin secretion. May alter absorption of concomitantly administered **oral medications** due to delayed gastric emptying.

Route/Dosage

Subcut (Adults): 0.6 mg once daily initially, may be ↑ at weekly intervals up to 1.8 mg/day.

Availability

Solution for subcutaneous injection: pre-filled, multi-dose pen that delivers doses of 0.6 mg, 1.2 mg, or 1.8 mg.

NURSING IMPLICATIONS

Assessment

● Observe patient taking concurrent insulin for signs and symptoms of hypoglycemic reactions (sweating, hunger, weakness, dizziness, tremor, tachycardia, anxiety).

● If thyroid nodules or elevated serum calcium are noted, patient should be referred to an endocrinologist.

● Monitor for pancreatitis (persistent severe abdominal pain, sometimes radiating to the back, with or without vomiting). If pancreatitis is suspected, discontinue liraglutide; if confirmed, do not restart liraglutide.

● *Lab Test Considerations:* Monitor serum HbA₁c periodically during therapy to evaluate effectiveness.

Potential Nursing Diagnoses

Imbalanced nutrition: more than body requirements (Indications)

Noncompliance (Patient/Family Teaching)

Implementation

● Patients stabilized on a diabetic regimen who are exposed to stress, fever, trauma, infection, or surgery may require administration of insulin.

● **Subcut:** Administer once daily at any time of the day, without regard to food. Inject into abdomen, thigh, or upper arm. Solution should be clear and colorless; do not administer solutions that are discolored or contain particulate matter.

● Initial dose of 0.6 mg/day is ↑ after 1 wk to 1.2 mg/day. If glycemic control is not acceptable, ↑ to 1.8 mg/day. Available in a prefilled pen without needle; patient may require Rx for needles.

● *First Time Use for Each New Pen—* Follow manufacturer's instructions only once with each new pen or if pen is dropped.

Patient/Family Teaching

● Instruct patient on use of *Victoza* pen and to take liraglutide as directed. Pen should never be shared between patients, even if needle is changed. Store pen in refrigerator; do not freeze. After initial use, pen may be stored at room temperature or refrigerated up to 30 days. Keep pen cap on when not in use. Protect from excessive heat and sunlight. Remove and safely discard needle after each injection and store pen without needle attached. Advise patient to read the *Patient Medication Guide* before starting liraglutide and with each Rx refill.

● Inform patient that nausea is the most common side effect, but usually ↓ s over time.

● Explain to patient that this medication controls hyperglycemia but does not cure diabetes. Therapy is long-term.

● Review signs of hypoglycemia and hyperglycemia with patient. If hypoglycemia occurs, advise patient to take a glass of orange juice or 2–3 tsp of sugar, honey, or corn syrup dissolved in water and notify health care professional.

- Encourage patient to follow prescribed diet, medication, and exercise regimen to prevent hypoglycemic or hyperglycemic episodes.
- Instruct patient in proper testing of serum glucose and ketones. These tests should be closely monitored during periods of stress or illness, and health care professional should be notified if significant changes occur.
- Advise patient to tell health care professional what medications they are taking and to avoid taking new Rx, OTC, vitamins, or herbal products without consulting health care professional.
- Advise patient to notify discontinue liraglutide and health care professional immediately if signs of pancreatitis occur.
- Inform patient of risk of benign and malignant thyroid C-cell tumors. Advise patient to notify health care professional if symptoms of thyroid tumors (lump in neck, hoarseness, trouble swallowing, shortness of breath) occur.
- Insulin is the preferred method of controlling blood glucose during pregnancy. Counsel female patients to notify health care professional if pregnancy is planned or suspected or if breastfeeding.
- Advise patient to inform health care professional of medication regimen before treatment or surgery.
- Advise patient to carry a form of sugar (sugar packets, candy) and identification describing disease process and medication regimen at all times.
- Emphasize the importance of routine follow-up exams.

Evaluation/Desired Outcomes

- Improved glycemic control.

lurasidone
(loo-**ras**-i-done)
Latuda

Classification
Thera: antipsychotics
Pharm: benzoisothiazole

Pregnancy Category B

Indications

Treatment of schizophrenia.

Action

Effect may mediated via effects on central dopamine Type 2 (D_2) and serotonin Type 2 ($5HT_{2A}$) receptor antagonism. **Therapeutic Effects:** ↓ schizophrenic behavior.

Pharmacokinetics

Absorption: 9–19% absorbed following oral administration.
Distribution: Unknown.
Protein Binding: >99%.
Metabolism and Excretion: Mostly metabolized by the CYP3A4 enzyme system. Two metabolites are pharmacologically active; 80% eliminated in feces, 8% in urine primarily as metabolites.
Half-life: 18 hr.

TIME/ACTION PROFILE

ROUTE	ONSET	PEAK	DURATION
PO	unknown	1–3 hr*	24 hr

*Blood level.

Contraindications/Precautions

Contraindicated in: Hypersensitivity.
Use Cautiously in: Renal/hepatic impairment (dose adjustment recommended for CCr of 10 mL/min–<50 mL/min or Child-Pugh Class B and C); History of suicide attempt; Diabetes mellitus; Overheating/dehydration (may ↑ risk of serious adverse reactions); History of leukopenia or previous drug-induced leukopenia/neutropenia; Geri: ↑ risk of seizures; elderly patients with dementia-related psychoses (↑ risk of cerebrovascular adverse reactions); use cautiously in elderly females (↑ risk of tardive dyskinesia); OB: Use in pregnancy only if potential benefit justifies potential risk to fetus; Lactation: breastfeeding should only be considered if potential benefit justifies risk to child; Pedi: Safe and effective use in children has not been established.

Adverse Reactions/Side Effects

CNS: NEUROLEPTIC MALIGNANT SYNDROME, SEIZURES, <u>akathisia</u>, <u>drowsiness</u>, <u>parkinsonism</u>, agitation, anxiety, cognitive/motor impairment, dizziness, dystonia, tardive dyskinesia. **EENT:** blurred vision. **CV:** bradycardia, orthostatic hypotension, syncope, tachycardia. **GI:** <u>nausea</u>, esophageal dysmotility. **Derm:** pruritus, rash. **Endo:** hyperglycemia, hyperprolactinemia. **Hemat:** AGRANULOCYTOSIS, anemia, leukopenia. **Metab:** dyslipidemia, weight gain.

Interactions

Drug-Drug: Strong inhibitors of the CYP3A4 enyzme system, including **ketoconazole**; ↑ blood levels and risk of adverse reactions; concurrent use should be avoided. **Moderate inhibitors of the CYP3A4 enzyme system**, including **diltiazem**, ↑ blood levels; if used concurrently dose of lurasidone should not exceed 40 mg/day. **Strong inducers of the CYP3A4 enzyme system**, including **rifampin** ↓ blood levels and effectiveness; concurrent use should be avoided. ↑ sedation may occur with other **CNS depressants**, including **alcohol**, **sedative/hypnotics**, **opioids**, some **antidepressants** and **antihistamines**.

Route/Dosage

PO (Adults): 40 mg once daily, not to exceed 80 mg once daily *Concurrent use of moderate CYP3A4 inhibitors*— dose should not exceed 40 mg once daily.

Renal Impairment

PO (Adults): *CCr of 10 mL/min – <50 mL/min*— dose should not exceed 40 mg once daily.

Hepatic Impairment

PO (Adults): *Child-Pugh Class B and C*— dose should not exceed 40 mg once daily.

Availability

Tablets : 40 mg, 80 mg.

NURSING IMPLICATIONS

Assessment

- Monitor patient's mental status (orientation, mood, behavior) before and periodically during therapy.
- Assess weight and BMI initially and throughout therapy.
- Monitor mood changes. Assess for suicidal tendencies, especially during early therapy. Restrict amount of drug available to patient.
- Monitor blood pressure (sitting, standing, lying down) and pulse before and frequently during initial dose titration. May cause tachycardia and orthostatic hypotension. If hypotension occurs, dose may need to be ↓.
- Observe patient when administering medication to ensure medication is swallowed and not hoarded or cheeked.
- Monitor patient for onset of extrapyramidal side effects (*akathisia*—restlessness; *dystonia*—muscle spasms and twisting motions; or *pseudoparkinsonism*—mask-like face, rigidity, tremors, drooling, shuffling gait, dysphagia). Report these symptoms; reduction of dose or discontinuation may be necessary. Trihexyphenidyl or benztropine may be used to control symptoms.
- Monitor for tardive dyskinesia (involuntary rhythmic movement of mouth, face, and extremities). Report immediately; may be irreversible.
- Monitor for development of neuroleptic malignant syndrome (fever, respiratory distress, tachycardia, seizures, diaphoresis, hypertension or hypotension, pallor, tiredness). Notify health care professional immediately if these symptoms occur.
- Monitor for symptoms of hyperglycemia (polydipsia, polyuria, polyphagia, weakness) periodically during therapy.
- *Lab Test Considerations:* May cause ↑ serum prolactin levels.
- May cause ↑ CPK.

- Obtain fasting blood glucose and cholesterol levels initially and periodically during therapy.
- Monitor CBC frequently during initial mo of therapy in patients with pre-existing or history of low WBC. May cause leukopenia, neutropenia, or agranulocytosis. Discontinue therapy if this occurs.

Potential Nursing Diagnoses
Risk for self-directed violence (Indications)
Disturbed thought process (Indications)
Risk for injury (Side Effects)

Implementation
- **PO:** Administer once daily with food.

Patient/Family Teaching
- Instruct patient to take medication as directed.
- Inform patient of the possibility of extrapyramidal symptoms. Instruct patient to report these symptoms immediately to health care professional.
- Advise patient to change positions slowly to minimize orthostatic hypotension.
- May cause drowsiness and cognitive and motor impairment. Caution patient to avoid driving or other activities requiring alertness until response to medication is known.
- Advise patient and family to notify health care professional if thoughts about suicide or dying, attempts to commit suicide; new or worse depression; new or worse anxiety; feeling very agitated or restless; panic attacks; trouble sleeping; new or worse irritability; acting aggressive; being angry or violent; acting on dangerous impulses; an extreme ↑ in activity and talking, other unusual changes in behavior or mood occur.
- Advise patient to avoid extremes in temperature; this drug impairs body temperature regulation.
- Caution patient to avoid concurrent use of alcohol, other CNS depressants, and OTC medications or herbal products without consulting health care professional.
- Advise female patients to notify health care professional if pregnancy is

planned or suspected, or if breastfeeding or planning to breastfeed.
- Advise patient to notify health care professional of medication regimen before treatment or surgery.
- Instruct patient to notify health care professional promptly if sore throat, fever, unusual bleeding or bruising, rash, or tremors occur.
- Emphasize the importance of routine follow up exams to monitor side effects and continued participation in psychotherapy to improve coping skills.

Evaluation/Desired Outcomes
- ↓ in symptoms of schizophrenia (delusions, hallucinations, social withdrawal, flat, blunted affects).

---

ofatumumab
(oh-fa-**too**-moo-mab)
Azerra

Classification
Thera: antineoplastics
Pharm: monoclonal antibodies

Pregnancy Category C

Indications
Chronic lymphocytic leukemia (CLL) refractory to fludarabine and alemtuzumab.

Action
A monoclonal antibody that specifically binds to CD20 molecule found on the surface of B lymphocytes, resulting in B-cell lysis. **Therapeutic Effects:** ↓ numbers of leukemic cells in CLL.

Pharmacokinetics
Absorption: IV administration results in complete bioavailability.
Distribution: Unknown.
Metabolism and Excretion: Unknown.
Half-life: 14 days (range: 2.3–61.5 days).

TIME/ACTION PROFILE

ROUTE	ONSET	PEAK	DURATION
IV	end of infusion	unknown	7 days

Contraindications/Precautions

Contraindicated in: None noted.
Use Cautiously in: History of hepatitis B infection (may reactivate); OB: Use during pregnancy only if potential benefit to mother justifies potential risk to fetus; Lactation: Use cautiously during lactation; Pedi: safe and effectiveness in children has not been established.

Adverse Reactions/Side Effects

CNS: weakness. **CV:** peripheral edema. **GI:** INTESTINAL OBSTRUCTION, REACTIVATION OF HEPATITIS B. **Derm:** sweating. **Hemat:** anemia, neutropenia, thrombocytopenia. **MS:** back pain, muscle spasm. **Neuro:** PROGRESSIVE MULTIFOCAL LEUKOENCEPHALOPATHY (PML). **Misc:** INFECTIONS, INFUSION REACTIONS, chills, fever.

Interactions

Drug-Drug: May ↓ antibody response to and ↑ risk of adverse reactions from **live-virus vaccines**.

Route/Dosage

IV (Adults): 300 mg initial initially, followed 1 wk later by 2000 mg weekly for 7 doses, followed 4 wk later by 2000 mg every 4 wk for 4 doses (total regimen is 12 doses).

Availability

Solution for IV administration (requires further dilution): 100 mg/5 mL vial.

NURSING IMPLICATIONS

Assessment

● Monitor for infusion reactions (bronchospasm, dyspnea, laryngeal edema, pulmonary edema, flushing, hypertension, hypotension, syncope, cardiac ischemia/infarction, back pain, abdominal pain, pyrexia, rash, urticaria, and angioedema); may occur more frequently with first 2 infusions. Institute medical management for severe infusion reactions. Interrupt infusion for infusion reactions of any severity. For Grade 4 reactions, do not resume infusion. For Grade 1, 2, or 3, if infusion re-

action resolves or remains less than or equal to Grade 2, resume infusion at one-half of previous infusion rate if Grade 1 or 2, or at a rate of 12 mL/hr if Grade 3. After resuming, infusion rate may be ↑ as described under rate, as tolerated.

● Monitor for signs of progressive multifocal leukoencephlopathy (PML) (new onset or changes in pre-existing neurological signs and symtoms). Initiate evaluation for PML (neurological consultation, brain MRI, lumbar puncture) if signs occur. Discontinue ofatumumab if PML is suspected.

● Screen patients at high risk for hepatitis B virus (HBV) infection before initiating therapy. Monitor carriers of HBV for clinical and laboratory signs during and for 6–12 months following discontinuation of therapy. Discontinue ofatumumab in patients who develop viral hepatitis or reactivation of viral hepatitis and institute appropriate treatment.

● **Lab Test Considerations:** Monitor CBC and platelet counts regularly during therapy and ↑ frequency of monitoring in patients who develop Grade 3 or 4 cytopenias. May cause prolonged (≥1 wk) severe neutropenia and thrombocytopenia.

Potential Nursing Diagnoses

Activity intolerance

Implementation

● Premedicate 30 min-2 hr prior to each dose with acetaminophen PO 1000 mg, PO or IV antihistamine (cetirizine 10 mg or equivalent), and IV corticosteroid (prednisolone 100 mg or equivalent). Do not reduce corticosteroid dose for Doses 1, 2, and 9. Corticosteroid dose may be reduced for doses 3–8 and 10–12. *Doses 3–8:* Gradually reduce corticosteroid dose with each infusion if a reaction ≥Grade 3 did not occur with preceeding does. *Doses 10–12:* Administer prednisolone 50–100 mg or equivalent if a reaction ≥Grade 3 did not occur with dose 9.

IV Administration

- **Intermittent Infusion: *Diluent:*** Dilute all doses in 1000 mL of 0.9% NaCl in a polyolefin bag*For 300 mg dose:* Withdraw and discard 15 mL from 0.9% NaCl bag. Withdraw 5 mL from each of 3 ofatumumab vials and add to 0.9% NaCl bag. *For 2000 mg dose:* Withdraw and discard 100 mL from 0.9% NaCl bag. Withdraw 5 mL from each of 20 ofatumumab vials and add to 0.9% NaCl bag. Do not shake; mix diluted solution by gentle inversion. Solution is colorless and may contain a small amount of visible translucent-to-white, amorphous particles; do not administer if discolored, cloudy, or if foreign matter is present Refrigerate solution, do not freeze; protect vials from light. Start infusion within 12 hr of preparation; discard after 24 hr. ***Rate:*** Administer through in-line filter supplied with medication using an infusion pump and PVC infusion set. Flush IV line with 0.9% NaCl before and after each dose. Do not administer as a IV push or bolus. Initiate infusion for *Dose 1* at 3.6 mg/hr (12 mL/hr), *Dose 2* at 24 mg/hr (12 mL/hr), *Doses 3–12* at 50 mg/hr (25 mL/hr). Rate for *Doses 1 and 2* may be ↑ every 30 min to 25, 50, 100, and 200 mL/hr if no infusional toxicity occurs. Rate for *Doses 3–12* may be ↑ every 30 min to 50, 100, 200, and 400 mL/hr if no infusional toxicity occurs.
- **Y-Site Incompatibility:** Do not mix with or infuse with other products.

Patient/Family Teaching

- Explain the purpose of ofatumumab to patient and caregiver.
- Advise patient to avoid live viral vaccines during therapy.
- Advise patient to notify health care professional immediately if signs and symptoms of infusion reactions (fever, chills, rash, breathing problems) occur within 24 hr of infusion or if bleeding, bruising, petechiae, pallor, worsening weakness, fatigue, cough, infection, confusion, dizziness, loss of balance, difficulty talking or walking, vision problems, yellow discoloration of skin

or eyes, new or worsening abdominal pain or nausea occur.
- Advise female patients to notify health care professional if pregnancy is planned or suspected or if breastfeeding.
- Emphasize the need for periodic blood count monitoring.

Evaluation/Desired Outcomes

- ↓ numbers of leukemic cells in CLL.

---

pegloticase
(peg-**loe**-ti-kase)
Krystexxa

Classification
Thera: antigout agents
Pharm: enzymes

Pregnancy Category C

Indications

Treatment of chronic gout in adults who have not responded to/cannot tolerate xanthine oxidase inhibitors, including allopurinol.

Action

Consists of recombinant uricase covalently bonded to monomethoxypoly(ethylene glycol) [mPEG]; uricase catalyzes the oxidation of uric acid to allantoin, a water soluble byproduct that is readily excreted in urine. **Therapeutic Effects:** ↓ serum uric acid levels with resultant ↓ in attacks of gout and its sequelae.

Pharmacokinetics

Absorption: IV administration results in complete bioavailability.
Distribution: Unknown.
Metabolism and Excretion: Unknown.
Half-life: Unknown.

TIME/ACTION PROFILE (effects on serum uric acid)

ROUTE	ONSET	PEAK	DURATION
IV	rapid	within 24 hr	>300 hr

Contraindications/Precautions

Contraindicated in: ⚠ Glucose-6–phosphate dehydrogenase (G6–PD) deficiency (risk of hemolysis and methemoglobinemia); Lactation: Breastfeeding is not recommended.

Use Cautiously in: Congestive heart failure (may ↑ risk of exacerbation); Retreatment after a drug-free interval (↑ risk of allergic reactions, monitor carefully); Geri: Elderly patients may be more sensitive to drug effects; OB: Use during pregnancy only if clearly needed; Pedi: Safe and effective use in children <18 yr not established.

Adverse Reactions/Side Effects

CV: chest pain. **EENT:** nasopharyngitis. **GI:** nausea, constipation, vomiting. **Derm:** contusion/ecchymoses. **Metab:** gout flare. **Misc:** allergic reactions including ANAPHYLAXIS, INFUSION REACTIONS.

Interactions

Drug-Drug: May interfere with the action of other **PEG-containing therapies**.

Route/Dosage

IV (Adults): 8 mg every two wk.

Availability

Injection for IV infusion (requires dilution): 8 mg/1 mL.

NURSING IMPLICATIONS

Assessment

- Monitor for joint pain and swelling. Gout flares frequently occur upon initiation of therapy, but do not require discontinuation. Administer prophylactic doses of colchicine or an NSAID at least 1 wk before and concurrently during the first 6 mo of therapy.
- Monitor for signs and symptoms of anaphylaxis (wheezing, peri-oral or lingual edema, hemodynamic instability, rash, urticaria) during and following infusion. May occur with any infusion, including initial infusion; usually occurs with 2 hrs of infusion. However, delayed reactions have been reported. Risk is higher in patients with uric acid level >6 m g/dL.
- Monitor for infusion reactions (rash, redness of skin, dyspnea, flushing, chest

discomfort, chest pain) during and periodically after infusion. If infusion reaction occurs, slow or stop infusion; restart at slower rate. If severe reaction occurs, discontinue infusion and treat as needed. Risk is greater in patients who have lost therapeutic response. Monitor patient for at least 1 hr following infusion.

- *Lab Test Considerations:* Monitor serum uric acid levels prior to infusion. Consider discontinuing therapy if levels ↑ to >6 m g/dL, especially if 2 consecutive levels are >6 m g/dL.

Potential Nursing Diagnoses

Chronic pain (Indications)

Implementation

- Premedicate patient with antihistamines and corticosteroids prior to infusion to minimize risk of anaphylaxis and infusion reaction. Administer in a setting with professionals prepared to manage anaphylaxis and infusion reactions.

IV Administration

- **Intermittent Infusion:** Withdraw 1 mL of pegloticase from vial and inject into 250 mL bag of NaCl; discard unused portion. Invert bag several times to mix; do not shake. Solution is clear and colorless; do not administer solutions that are discolored or contain a precipitate. Solution is stable for 4 hrs if refrigerated or at room temperature. Store in refrigerator and protect from light; do not freeze. Allow solution to reach room temperature before administering; do not use artificial heating. *Rate:* Infuse over 120 min.
- **Additive Incompatibility:** Do not mix with other medications.

Patient/Family Teaching

- Explain purpose of pegloticase to patient. Instruct patient to read *Medication Guide* before starting therapy before each infusion.
- Advise patient to notify health care professional immediately if signs of anaphylaxis or infusion reaction occur.

- ☒ Advise patient not to take pegloticase if they have G6PD deficiency.
- Inform patient that gout flares may initially ↑ at the start of pegloticase. Advise patient to not to stop therapy but to take medication (colchicine, NSAID) to reduce flares regularly for the first few mo of pegloticase therapy.
- Advise female patient to notify health care professional if pregnancy is planned or suspected or if breastfeeding.

Evaluation/Desired Outcomes
- ↓ in uric acid levels with resultant improvement in gout symptoms in patients with chronic gout.

---

pentosan (pen-toe-san)
Elmiron

Classification
Thera: agents for interstitial cystitis
Pharm: heparin-like compounds

Pregnancy Category B

Indications
Management symptoms (bladder pain/discomfort) of chronic interstitial cystitis (IC).

Action
Adheres to uroepithelium, providing a protective barrier against irritating solutes in urine. Has anticoagulant and fibrinolytic properties. **Therapeutic Effects:** ↓ pain and discomfort in chronic IC.

Pharmacokinetics
Absorption: 6% absorbed following oral administrations.
Distribution: Distributes into uroepithelium of the genitourinary tract with less found in liver, spleen, lung, skin, periosteum and bone marrow.
Metabolism and Excretion: Metabolized by saturable enzyme systems in liver, spleen and kidney. Majority (58–84%) excreted in feces as unchanged (unabsorbed drug). Metabolites of absorbed drug

are renally excreted; minimal renal excretion of unchanged drug.
Half-life: 27 hr.

TIME/ACTION PROFILE (↓ symptoms)

ROUTE	ONSET	PEAK	DURATION
PO	within 4 wk-6 mos	unknown	unknown

Contraindications/Precautions
Contraindicated in: Hypersensitivity.
Use Cautiously in: Underlying coagulopathy, concurrent medications that ↑ bleeding risk, history of aneurysms. thrombocytopenia, hemophilia, GI ulceration/bleeding, polyps, diverticula; History of heparin-induced thrombocytopenia; risk of bleeding may be ↑ ; Hepatic insufficiency; OB: Use in pregnancy only if clearly needed; Lactation: Use cautiously in breastfeeding women; Pedi: safe and effective use in children <16 yr has not been established.

Adverse Reactions/Side Effects
CNS: dizziness, headache. **EENT:** epistaxis. **GI:** abdominal pain, diarrhea, dyspepsia, gum bleeding, ↑ liver enzymes, nausea, rectal bleeding. **Derm:** alopecia, ecchymosis, rash. **Hemat:** bleeding, ↑ bleeding time.

Interactions
Drug-Drug: Concurrent use of **coumarin anticoagulants**, **heparins**, **t-PA**, **streptokinase**, high dose **aspirin**, or **NSAIDs** may ↑ risk of bleeding.

Route/Dosage
PO (Adults): 100 mg three times daily.

Availability
Capsules: 100 mg.

NURSING IMPLICATIONS
Assessment
- Assess pain intensity, frequency, and duration in patient with interstitial cystitis.
- **Lab Test Considerations:** Doses of <1200 mg/day are unlikely to affect PT or PTT.
- May cause liver function abnormalities.

- May rarely cause anemia, ↑ PT, ↑ PTT, leukopenia, and thrombocytopenia.

Potential Nursing Diagnoses
Chronic pain (Indications)

Implementation
- **PO:** Administer on an empty stomach 3 times daily, at least 1 hr before or 2 hrs after meals.

Patient/Family Teaching
- Instruct patient to take pentosan as directed, taking no more or no more frequently than prescribed.
- Advise patient to notify health care professional if surgery, anticoagulant therapy (warfarin, heparin), or therapy with high doses of aspirin or NSAIDs is planned.
- Advise patient to notify health care professional if pregnancy is planned or suspected or if breastfeeding.

Evaluation/Desired Outcomes
- ↓ in pain and discomfort of interstitial cystitis. Reassess after 3 months of therapy. If no improvement but no limiting adverse events are present, may be continued for 3 more mo.

---

polidocanol
(po-li-**doe**-ka-nole)
Ascelera

Classification
Thera: Sclerosing agents

Pregnancy Category C

Indications
Treatment of uncomplicated spider veins (varicose veins ≤1 mm in diameter) and uncomplicated reticular veins (varicose veins 1 to 3 mm in diameter) in legs.

Action
Causes local endothelial damage following intravenous administration, followed by platelet aggregation and attachment to the venous wall, resulting in a dense network of platelets, cellular debris, and fibrin, which occludes the vein. This is followed by replacement with connective fibrous tissue. **Therapeutic Effects:** Improved appearance of spider/reticular veins.

Pharmacokinetics
Absorption: Local IV administration results in low systemic blood levels.
Distribution: Action is primarily local.
Metabolism and Excretion: Unkown.
Half-life: 1.5 hr.

TIME/ACTION PROFILE (vessel occlusion)

ROUTE	ONSET	PEAK	DURATION
IV	rapid	3–6 wk	unknown

Contraindications/Precautions
Contraindicated in: Known allergy; Known thromboembolic disease; OB: Should not be used during pregnancy; Lactation: Avoid breastfeeding.
Use Cautiously in: Pedi: Safe and effective use in children has not been established.

Adverse Reactions/Side Effects
Local: mild injection site reactions.
Misc: allergic reactions including ANA-PHYLAXIS.

Interactions
Drug-Drug: None noted.

Route/Dosage
Local, IV (Adults): *Spider veins*— 0.1–0.3 mL of 0.5% solution for each injection into each varicose vein; *Reticular veins*— 0.1–0.3 mL of 1% solution for each injection into each varicose vein. Not to exceed 10 mL/treatment session.

Availability
Solution for local intravenous injection (contains ethanol): 5 mg/mL in 2 mL ampules (0.5%), 10 mg/mL in 2 mL ampules (1.0%).

NURSING IMPLICATIONS
Assessment
- Assess extent of spider and/or reticular veins in lower extremities.

🍁 = Canadian drug name. 🧬 = Genetic implication.
*CAPITALS indicates life-threatening; underlines indicate most frequent.

- Monitor for signs and symptoms of anaphylaxis (rash, pruritus, laryngeal edema, wheezing) for at least 15–20 min following administration.

Potential Nursing Diagnoses
Activity intolerance (Indications)
Disturbed body image (Indications)

Implementation

IV Administration

- **Direct IV:** Administer undiluted. Using a fine-gauge (26 or 30 gauge) needle, insert needle tangentially into affected vein and inject solution slowly while needle is still in vein. Apply only gently pressure during injection to prevent vein rupture. If repeated treatments are needed, separate by 1–2 wks.
- Inadvertent perivascular injection may cause pain. If severe, inject local anesthetic.
- Intra-arterial injection can cause severe necrosis, ischemia, or gangrene; consult a vascular surgeon immediately if this occurs.
- Following injection, apply compression via stocking or bandage to reduce risk of deep vein thrombisis. After treatment session, encourage patient to walk for 15–20 minutes.

Patient/Family Teaching

- Instruct patient to wear compression stockings or support hose on treated legs continuously for 2–3 days and for 2–3 wks during daytime. Compression stockings or support hose should be thigh high or knee high depending on area treated.
- Advise patient to walk for 15–20 min immediately after procedure and daily for next few days.
- Advise patient to avoid heavy exercise, sunbathing, long plane flights, and hot baths or sauna for 2–3 days following treatment.
- Advise patient to notify health care professional if pregnancy is planned or suspected or if breastfeeding.

Evaluation/Desired Outcomes

- ↓ in size and visibility of spider and/or uncomplicated reticular veins in lower extremities.

roflumilast
(row-**floo**-mi-last)
Daliresp

Classification
Thera: agents for COPD
Pharm: phosphodiesterase inhibitors

Pregnancy Category C

Indications
To ↓ the risk of exacerbations in severe COPD patients that have a history of chronic bronchitis with exacerbations.

Action
Roflumilast and one active metabolite (roflumilast N-oxide) act as selective inhibitors of phosphodiesterase 4 (PDE4), responsible for breaking down 3', 5'-adenosine monophosphate (cAMP). Resulting intracellular accumulation of cAMP in lung tissue. Reduces cells (neutrophils, eosinophils and total cells) in sputum. **Therapeutic Effects:** ↓ exacerbations in COPD patients.

Pharmacokinetics
Absorption: Well absorbed following oral administration.
Distribution: Parent drug and metabolites probably enter breast milk.
Protein Binding: *Roflumilast*—99%; *roflumilast N-oxide*—97%.
Metabolism and Excretion: Mostly metabolized (87.5%), primarily by CYP3A4 and CYP1A2 enzyme systems One metabolite, roflumilast N-oxide in pharmacologically active. Inactive metabolites excreted in urine.
Half-life: *Roflumilast*—17 hr; *roflumilast N-oxide*—30 hr.

TIME/ACTION PROFILE (blood levels)

ROUTE	ONSET	PEAK	DURATION
PO	unknown	1 (4–13†)	24 hr

†For roflumilast N-oxide.

Contraindications/Precautions

Contraindicated in: Acute broncho-spasm; Moderate to severe hepatic impairment; Concurrent use of strong inducers of CYP3A4 and CYP1A2 enzyme system; Lactation: Avoid breast-feeding.

Use Cautiously in: History of depression/suicidal thoughts; OB: Use only if potential maternal benefit justifies potential risk to the fetus; Pedi: Safe and effective use in children has not been established.

Adverse Reactions/Side Effects

CNS: SUICIDAL THOUGHTS, anxiety, depression, dizziness, headache, insomnia. **GI:** diarrhea, abdominal pain, ↓ appetite, dyspepsia, gastritis, nausea, vomiting. **Metab:** weight loss. **MS:** muscle spasms. **Neuro:** tremor.

Interactions

Drug-Drug: Strong inducers of the CYP3A4 and CYP1A2 enzyme systems, including **rifampicin**, **phenobarbital**, **carbamazepine**, and **phenytoin** ↓ blood levels and effectiveness; concurrent use should be avoided. Blood levels and risk of adverse reactions ↑ by concurrent use of **inhibitors of the CYP3A4 enzyme system** and **dual inhibitors of the CP3A4 and CYP1A2 enzyme systems** including **erythromycin**, **ketoconazole**, **fluvoxamine**, **enoxacin**, and **cimetidine**. **Gestodene** and **ethinyl estradiol** may also ↑ levels and risk of adverse reactions; risk should be considered.

Route/Dosage

PO (Adults): 500 mcg once daily.

Availability

Tablets: 500 mcg.

NURSING IMPLICATIONS

Assessment

- Assess respiratory status periodically during therapy.
- Monitor weight regularly. If unexplained or clinically significant weight loss occurs, evaluate weight loss and consider discontinuation of roflumilast.

- Assess mental status (orientation, mood, behavior) before and periodically during therapy. Assess for suicidal tendencies.

Potential Nursing Diagnoses

Ineffective airway clearance

Implementation

- **PO:** Administer without regard to food.

Patient/Family Teaching

- Instruct patient to take roflumilast as directed. Advise patient to read *Medication Guide* before starting therapy and with each Rx refill; new information may be available.
- Inform patient that roflumilast is not a bronchodilator and should not be used for treating sudden breathing problems.
- Advise patient to monitor weight regularly. If weight loss occurs, notify health care professional; may require discontinuation of therapy.
- Advise patient and family to notify health care professional if thoughts about suicide or dying, attempts to commit suicide, trouble sleeping, new or worse depression, new or worse anxiety, acting on dangerous impulses, or other unusual changes in behavior or mood occur.
- Instruct patient to notify health care professional of all Rx or OTC medications, vitamins, or herbal products being taken and to avoid concurrent use of Rx, OTC, and herbal products without consulting health care professional.
- Advise female patient to notify health care professional if pregnancy is planned or suspected or if breastfeeding.

Evaluation/Desired Outcomes

- ↓ in the number of flare-ups or the worsening of COPD symptoms (exacerbations).

---

romidepsin
(roe-mi-**dep**-sin)
ISTODAX

Classification
Thera: antineoplastics
Pharm: enzyme inhibitors

Pregnancy Category D

Indications
Treatment of cutaneous T-cell lymphoma (CTCL) that has not responded to at least one prior systemic therapy.

Action
Acts as an inhibitor of histone deacetylase (HDAC). HDACs modulate gene expression and transcription factors. Inhibition results in cell cycle arrest and apoptosis. **Therapeutic Effects:** ↓ extent and spread of CTCL.

Pharmacokinetics
Absorption: IV administration results in complete bioavailability.
Distribution: Unknown.
Protein Binding: 92–94%.
Metabolism and Excretion: Extensively metabolized, mostly by the CYP3A4 enzyme system.
Half-life: 3 hr.

TIME/ACTION PROFILE (response)

ROUTE	ONSET	PEAK	DURATION
IV	2 mos	4–6 mos	25–33 mos

Contraindications/Precautions
Contraindicated in: OB: Pregnancy (may cause fetal harm); Lactation: Avoid use.

Use Cautiously in: Congenital long QT syndrome, history of significant cardiovascular disease, concurrent anti-arrhythmics or other medications that cause significant QT prolongation (↑ risk of arrhythmias); Electrolyte abnormalities (correct magnesium and potassium abnormalities prior to use); Moderate to severe hepatic impairment or end-stage renal disease; Geri: Elderly patients may be more sensitive to drug effects; Pedi: Safe and effective use in children has not been established.

Adverse Reactions/Side Effects
CNS: fatigue. **CV:** ECG changes. **GI:** anorexia, nausea, vomiting. **Hemat:** ANEMIA, LEUKOPENIA, THROMBOCYTOPENIA.

Interactions
Drug-Drug: May ↑ risk of bleeding with **warfarin** or **NSAIDs**. May ↓ effectiveness of **estrogen-containing contraceptives** (competes with β-estradiol for binding to estrogen receptors). **Strong CYP3A4 inhibitors** including **ketoconazole, itraconazole, clarithromycin, atazanavir, indinavir, nefazodone, nelfinavir, ritonavir, saquinavir, telithromycin,** and **voriconazole** may ↑ levels and risk of toxicity; avoid concurrent use. **Strong CYP3A4 inducers** including **dexamethasone, carbamazepine, phenytoin, rifampin, rifabutin, rifapentine,** and **phenobarbital** may ↓ levels and effectiveness; avoid concurrent use. **Drugs that inhibit P-gp** including **amiodarone, atorvastatin, cyclosporine, dipyridamole, ketoconazole, nelfinavir, quinidine, quinine, reserpine, saquinavir, spironolactone, tacrolimus,** and **verapamil** may ↑ levels and the risk of toxicity; use cautiously.

Route/Dosage
IV (Adults): 14 mg/m² on days 1, 8 and 15 of a 28-day cycle, cycle may be repeated every 28 days depending on benefit and patient tolerance; dose may be ↓ to 10 mg/m² if adverse reactions occur.

Availability
Lyophilized powder for injection (requires reconstitution): 20 mg/vial (contains povidone; enclosed diluent contains propylene glycol and dehydrated alcohol).

NURSING IMPLICATIONS
Assessment
- Monitor blood pressure, pulse, respiratory rate, and temperature frequently during administration. Report significant changes.
- Monitor ECG and electrolytes at baseline and periodically during therapy. May cause T-wave and ST-segment changes.
- Monitor for bone marrow depression. Assess for bleeding (bleeding gums, bruising, petechiae, guaiac stools,

urine, and emesis) and avoid IM injections and taking rectal temperatures if platelet count is low. Apply pressure to venipuncture sites for 10 min. Assess for signs of infection during neutropenia. Anemia may occur. Monitor for ↑ fatigue, dyspnea, and orthostatic hypotension.

- Severe and protracted nausea and vomiting may occur. Administer antiemetics prior to therapy and routinely as indicated. Monitor amount of emesis and health care professional if emesis exceeds guidelines to prevent dehydration. *If Grade 2 or 3 nonhematologic toxicity occurs,* delay therapy until toxicity returns to ≤Grade 1 or baseline, then therapy may be restarted at 14 mg/m². *If Grade 3 toxicity recurs or Grade 4 toxicity occurs,* delay therapy until toxicity returns to ≤Grade 1 or baseline and permanently reduce dose to 10 mg/m². Discontinue therapy if Grade 3 or 4 toxicities recur after dose reduction.

- *Lab Test Considerations:* Ensure serum potassium and magnesium are within normal range before administration.

- Monitor CBC and differential prior to and periodically during therapy. May cause neutropenia or thrombocytopenia. Delay therapy until ANC ≥1.5 x 10⁹/L and/or platelet count ≥75 x 10⁹/L or baseline, then restart therapy at 14 mg/m². If Grade 4 febrile (≥38.5°C) neutropenia or thrombocytopenia that requires platelet transfusion occurs, delay therapy until ≤Grade 1 or baseline, and then permanently ↓ dose to 10 mg/m².

Potential Nursing Diagnoses
Risk for infection (Adverse Reactions)

Implementation
- *High Alert:* Fatalities have occurred with incorrect administration of chemotherapeutic agents. Before administering, clarify all ambiguous orders; double check single, daily, and course-of-therapy dose limits; have second practitioner independently double check original order, calculations and infusion pump settings. Clarify orders that do not include generic and brand names.

IV Administration

- Solution should be prepared in a biologic cabinet. Wear gloves, gown, and mask while handling medication. Discard IV equipment in specially designated containers (see Appendix L).

- **Intermittent Infusion:** Reconstitute each 10 mg vial with 2 mL of supplied diluent. Slowly inject diluent into vial. Swirl until no visible particles in solution. Solution is stable for 8 hrs at room temperature *Concentration:* 5 mg/mL. *Diluent:* Dilute further in 500 mL of 0.9% NaCl. Do not administer solution that is discolored or contains particulate matter. Dilutes solution is stable for 24 hrs at room temperature. *Rate:* Infuse over 4 hr.

Patient/Family Teaching
- Advise patient to read the *Patient Information* that comes with medication prior to each dose.

- Instruct patient to notify health care professional promptly if excessive nausea or vomiting, abnormal heartbeat, chest pain, shortness of breath, fever; sore throat; signs of infection; bleeding gums; bruising; petechiae; blood in stools, urine, or emesis; ↑ fatigue occurs. Caution patient to avoid crowds and persons with known infections. Instruct patient to use soft toothbrush and electric razor and to avoid falls. Caution patient not to drink alcoholic beverages or take medication containing aspirin or NSAIDs, because these may precipitate gastric bleeding.

- Instruct patient to notify health care professional of all Rx or OTC medications, vitamins, or herbal products being taken and consult health care professional before taking any new medications.

- Advise patient that this medication may have teratogenic effects. Non-hormonal contraception should be used during therapy. Advise patient to notify health care professional if pregnancy is planned or suspected or is breastfeeding.

• Emphasize the need for periodic lab tests to monitor for side effects.

Evaluation/Desired Outcomes
• ↓ extent and spread of CTCL.

---

rufinamide
(roo-**fin**-a-mide)
Banzol

Classification
Thera: anticonvulsants
Pharm: triazoles

Pregnancy Category C

Indications
Adjunctive treatment of seizures associated with Lennox-Gastaut syndrome in patients >4 yr.

Action
Although antiepileptic mechanism is unknown, rufinamide modulates the activity of sodium channels, prolonging the inactive state of the channel. **Therapeutic Effects:** ↓ incidence and severity of seizures associated with Lennox-Gastaut syndrome.

Pharmacokinetics
Absorption: 85% absorbed following oral administration; food enhances absorption.
Distribution: Evenly distributed between erythrocytes and plasma.
Metabolism and Excretion: Extensively metabolized; metabolites are primarily renaly excreted.
Half-life: 6–10 hr.

TIME/ACTION PROFILE

ROUTE	ONSET	PEAK	DURATION
PO	unknown	4–6 hr	12 hr

Contraindications/Precautions
Contraindicated in: Hypersensitivity; Familial short QT syndrome; Severe hepatic impairment.

Use Cautiously in: All patients (may ↑ risk of suicidal thoughts/behaviors); Mild to moderate hepatic impairment.

Adverse Reactions/Side Effects
CNS: SUICIDAL THOUGHTS, dizziness, fatigue, headache, somnolence. **EENT:** diplopia. **CV:** QT prolongation. **GI:** nausea, changes in appetite. **GU:** urinary frequency. **Derm:** rash. **Hemat:** anemia. **Neuro:** ataxia, coordination abnormalities, gait disturbances. **Misc:** MULTI-ORGAN HYPERSENSITIVITY REACTIONS, hypersensitivity reactions (↑ children).

Interactions
Drug-Drug: Potent inducers of the **CYP450 enzyme** including **carbamazepine**, **phenytoin**, **primidone**, and **phenobarbital** ↑ clearance and may ↓ blood levels. **Valproate** ↓ clearance and may ↑ blood levels; valproate should be started at a low dose in patients stabilized on rufinamide. In patients stabilized on valproate, rufinamide should be started at a low dose. May ↓ blood levels and effectiveness of **hormonal contraceptives**. May ↑ blood levels of **phenytoin**.

Route/Dosage
PO (Adults): 400–800 mg/day in two divided doses, ↑ by 400–800 mg every 2 days until a maximum daily dose of 3200 mg/day (1600 mg twice daily) is reached.
PO (Children ≥4 yr): 10 mg/kg/day in two divided doses, ↑ by 10 mg/kg every 2 days until a maximum daily dose of 45 mg/kg/day or 3200 mg/day given in 2 divided doses, whichever is less, is reached.

Availability
Tablets: 200 mg.

NURSING IMPLICATIONS
Assessment
• Assess location, duration, and characteristics of seizure activity. Institute seizure precautions.
• Monitor closely for notable changes in behavior that could indicate the emergence or worsening of suicidal thoughts or behavior or depression.
• *Lab Test Considerations:* May cause leukopenia, anemia, neutropenia, and thrombocytopenia.

Potential Nursing Diagnoses
Risk for injury (Indications)

Implementation
- **PO:** Administer with food. Tablets can be cut in half for dosing flexibility. Tablets may be administered as whole or half tablets, or crushed.

Patient/Family Teaching
- Instruct patient to take rufinamide around the clock, as directed. Medication should be gradually discontinued over by 25% every 2 days to prevent seizures. Advise patient to read the *Medication Guide* before starting therapy and with each Rx refill.
- May cause drowsiness, dizziness, ataxia, and incoordination. Caution patient to avoid driving or other activities requiring alertness until response to medication is known. Tell patient not to resume driving until physician gives clearance based on control of seizure disorder.
- Inform patients and families of risk of suicidal thoughts and behavior and advise that behavioral changes, emergency or worsening signs and symptoms of depression, unusual changes in mood, or emergence of suicidal thoughts, behavior, or thoughts of self-harm should be reported to health care professional immediately.
- Instruct patient to notify health care professional if signs of multiorgan hypersensitivity reactions (fever, rash, fatigue, jaundice, dark urine) occur.
- Advise patient to consult health care professional before taking other Rx, OTC, or herbal preparations and to avoid taking alcohol or other CNS depressants concurrently with rufinamide.
- Advise female patients to notify health care professional if pregnancy is planned or suspected or if breastfeeding. Use of rufinamide ↓ s effectiveness of oral contraceptives. Advise patient to use a nonhormonal method of contraception during therapy.

Evaluation/Desired Outcomes
- ↓ frequency and intensity of seizure activity.

---

sipuleucel (si-pu-loo-sel)
Provenge

Classification
Thera: antineoplastics
Pharm: autologous cellular immunotherapies

Indications
Asymptomatic/minimally symptomatic metastatic castrate resistant (hormone refractory) prostate cancer.

Action
Autologous immunotherapy produced by collecting peripheral mononuclear cells during leukapheresis. Cells include antigen presenting cells (APCs), which are activated during a culture period with prostatic acid phosphatase (PAP, an antigen found in prostatic cancer tissue) linked to granulocyte-macrophage colony-stimulating factor (GM-CSF, which activates immune cells). Induces an immune response against prostatic acid phosphatase. **Therapeutic Effects:** ↓ spread of prostate cancer.

Pharmacokinetics
Absorption: IV administration results in complete bioavailability.
Distribution: Unknown.
Metabolism and Excretion: Unknown.
Half-life: Unknown.

TIME/ACTION PROFILE

ROUTE	ONSET	PEAK	DURATION
IV	unknown	unknown	unknown

Contraindications/Precautions
Contraindicated in: None noted.
Use Cautiously in: Intended for autologous use only.

Adverse Reactions/Side Effects
CNS: <u>fatigue</u>, <u>headache</u>, dizziness, insomnia. **Resp:** dyspnea. **CV:** hypertension,

peripheral edema. **GI:** constipation, diarrhea, nausea, vomiting. **GU:** hematuria. **Derm:** flushing, rash, sweating. **Hemat:** anemia. **MS:** <u>back pain</u>, <u>joint pain</u>, extremity pain, muscle spasms, musculoskeletal pain. **Neuro:** paresthesia, tremor. **Misc:** <u>chills</u>, <u>fever</u>, acute infusion reactions, citrate toxicity.

Interactions

Drug-Drug: Concurrent use of **immunosuppressants** may alter safety/efficacy.

Route/Dosage

IV (Adults): One dose every two wk for a total of three doses.

Availability

Suspension for IV infusion: minimum of 50 million autologous CD54+ cells activated with PAP-GM-CSF suspended in 250 mL Lactated Ringer's Injection.

NURSING IMPLICATIONS

Assessment

- Monitor for signs of acute infusion reaction (fever, chills, dyspnea, hypoxia, bronchospasm, dizziness, nausea, vomiting, fatigue, headache, muscle aches, hypertension, tachycardia), especially patients with cardiac or pulmonary conditions. If signs occur, infusion may be slowed or interrupted, depending on severity of reaction. If infusion must be interrupted, do not resume if infusion bag will be at room temperature for >3 hrs. Monitor patient for at least 30 min following each infusion.

Potential Nursing Diagnoses

Deficient knowledge, related to medication regimen (Patient/Family Teaching)

Implementation

IV Administration

- Each infusion must be preceded by a leukaphresis procedure approximately 3 days prior. If patient is unable to receive an infusion, patient will need to undergo an additional leukaphresis procedure.
- Medication is not routinely tested for transmissible infectious diseases. Employ universal precautions in handling leukapheresis material or sipuleucel.
- Premedicate patient with acetaminophen and an antihistamine (diphenhydramine) 30 min prior to administration to minimize acute infusion reactions.
- Upon receipt of sipuleucel from manufacturer, open outer cardboard shipping box to verify product and patient-specific labels. Do not remove insulated container from shipping box, or open lid of insulated container, until patient is ready for infusion. Do not infuse until confirmation of product release has been received from manufacturer.
- Infusion must begin prior to expiration date and time. Do not infuse expired sipuleucel. Once infusion bag is removed from insulated container, infuse within 3 hrs; do not return to shipping container.
- **Intermittent Infusion:** Once patient is prepared for infusion and Cell Product Disposition Form has been received, remove infusion bag from insulated container, and inspect bag for leakage. Contents will be slightly cloudy, with cream-to-pink color. Gently mix and resuspend contents of bag, inspecting for clumps and clots. Small clumps should disperse with gentle manual mixing; do not administer if bag leaks or if clumps remain.
- Sipuleucel is solely for autologous use. Match patient's identity with the patient identifiers on the Cell Product Disposition Form and infusion bag. ***Rate:*** Infuse the entire volume of the bag over 60 min. Do not use a cell filter.

Patient/Family Teaching

- Explain the purpose of sipuleucel and the importance of maintaining all scheduled appointments, adhering to preparation instructions for leukaphresis procedure to patient.
- Inform patient that a central venous catheter may be required if adequate peripheral venous access is not available.
- Advise patient to notify health care professional if fever over 100°F, swelling or

redness around catheter site, pain at infusion or collection sites, symptoms of cardiac arrhythmia (chest pains, racing heart, irregular heartbeats), signs of acute infusion reaction, or persistent side effects occur.

- Instruct patient to notify health care professional of all Rx or OTC medications, vitamins, or herbal products, especially immunosuppressive agents, being taken and consult health care professional before taking any new medications.

Evaluation/Desired Outcomes

- ↓ in the spread of prostate cancer.

---

spinosad (spy-no-sad)
Natroba

Classification
Thera: pediculocides

Pregnancy Category B

Indications
Treatment of head lice in adults and children >4 yr.

Action
Causes neuronal hyperexcitation in insects, resulting paralysis and death of lice. **Therapeutic Effects:** Eradication of head lice.

Pharmacokinetics
Absorption: Undetectable systemic absorption follows topical use.
Distribution: Unknown.
Metabolism and Excretion: Unknown.
Half-life: Unknown.

TIME/ACTION PROFILE

ROUTE	ONSET	PEAK	DURATION
Topical	within min	unknown	unknown

Contraindications/Precautions
Contraindicated in: Pedi: Children <6 mos (↑ risk of benzyl alcohol absorption).

Use Cautiously in: OB: Use in pregnancy only if clearly needed; Lactation: use with caution; Pedi: Safe and effective use in children <4 yr not established.

Adverse Reactions/Side Effects
EENT: ocular erythema. **Local:** erythema.

Interactions
Drug-Drug: None noted.

Route/Dosage
Topical (Adults and Children >4 yr): Apply amount necessary to wet scalp, leave in place for 10 minutes, then rinse; may be repeated after 7 days if live lice are still seen.

Availability
Topical suspension: 0.9% in 120 mL bottles.

NURSING IMPLICATIONS

Assessment
- Assess scalp for presence of lice and their ova (nits) prior to and 1 wk after application of spinosad.

Potential Nursing Diagnoses
Impaired home maintenance (Indications)
Bathing/hygiene self-care deficit (Indications)

Implementation
- **Topical:** For topical application only.

Patient/Family Teaching
- Instruct patient/parent on correct application technique and not to change treatment without consulting health care professional. Use suspension in 1 or 2 treatments that are 1 wk apart. If live lice are seen 7 days after first application, repeat application. Shake bottle well. Cover face and eyes with a towel and keep eyes tightly closed. Use suspension only on dry scalp and dry hair. Completely cover scalp first, then apply outwards towards ends of hair. Use enough suspension to coat completely every single louse. Leave it on scalp for a full 10 min. Continue to keep eyes

covered to prevent dripping into eyes. Because all lice must be covered, help with application is advised. After 10 mins, completely rinse suspension from hair and scalp with warm water. Wash hands after application. Hair may be shampooed any time after treatment.

- Instruct patient to avoid swallowing suspension or getting suspension in eyes. If suspension gets in eyes, flush eyes thoroughly with water.
- Advise patient/parent that others residing in the home should be examined for lice.
- Instruct patient/parent on methods of preventing re-infestation. All clothes, including outdoor apparel and household linens, should be machine-washed using very hot water and dried for at least 20 min in a hot dryer. Soak brushes and combs in hot (130° F), soapy water for 5–10 min. Remind patient that brushes and combs should not be shared. Shampoo wigs and hairpieces. Vacuum rugs and upholstered furniture. Wash toys in hot, soapy water. Items that cannot be washed should be sealed in a plastic bag for 2 wks.
- If patient is a child, instruct parents to notify school nurse or day care center so that classmates and playmates can be checked.
- Advise female patient to notify health care professional if pregnancy is planned or suspected, or if breastfeeding. Lactating women may choose to pump and discard breast milk for 8 hrs after use to avoid infant ingestion.

Evaluation/Desired Outcomes

- Absence of lice and nits.

---

telavancin (tel-a-**van**-sin)
Vibativ

Classification
Thera: anti-infectives
Pharm: lipoglycopeptides

Pregnancy Category C

Indications

Treatment of complicated skin/skin structure infections caused by susceptible bacteria.

Action

Inhibits bacterial cell wall synthesis by interfering with the polymerization and cross-linking of peptidoglycan. **Therapeutic Effects:** Bactericidal action against susceptible organisms. **Spectrum:** Active against *Staphylococcus aureus* (including methicillin-susceptible and -resistant strains), *Streptococcus pyogenes*, *Streptococcus agalactiae*, *Streptococcus anginosus* (including *S. anginosus*, *S. intermedius*, and *S. constellatus*), and *Enterococcus faecalis* (vancomycin-susceptible strains only).

Pharmacokinetics

Absorption: IV administration results in complete bioavailability.
Distribution: Penetrates blister fluid.
Metabolism and Excretion: Metabolism is not known; 76% excreted unchanged in urine <1% in feces.
Half-life: 8 hr.

TIME/ACTION PROFILE

ROUTE	ONSET	PEAK	DURATION
IV	unknown	end of infusion	24 hr

Contraindications/Precautions

Contraindicated in: Congenital long QT syndrome, known prolongation of the QTc interval, uncompensated heart failure, or severe left ventricular hypertrophy (risk of fatal arrhythmias); OB: do not use during pregnancy unless potential maternal benefit outweighs potential risk to fetus.
Use Cautiously in: Renal impairment (efficacy may be reduced; dose reduction recommended for CCr ≤50 mL/min); Geri: Consider age-related ↓ in renal function, adjust dose accordingly (↑ risk of adverse renal reactions); Lactation: Use cautiously during breastfeeding; Pedi: Safety and effectiveness in children have not been established.

Adverse Reactions/Side Effects

CNS: dizziness. **CV:** QTc prolongation. **GI:** PSEUDOMEMBRANOUS COLITIS, taste disturbance, nausea, vomiting, abdominal pain. **GU:** foamy urine, nephrotoxicity. **Misc:** infusion reactions.

Interactions

Drug-Drug: Concurrent use of other **medications known to prolong QTc interval** may ↑ risk of arrhythmias. Concurrent use of **NSAIDs**, **ACE inhibitors**, and **loop diuretics** may ↑ risk of adverse renal effects.

Route/Dosage

IV (Adults): 10 mg/kg ever 24 hr for 7–14 days.

Renal Impairment

IV (Adults): *CCr 30–50 mL/min*—7.5 mg/kg every 24 hr; *CCr 10–≤30 mL/min*—10 mg/kg every 48 hr.

Availability

Sterile lyophilized powder for IV use (requires reconstitution): 250 mg vial, 750 mg vial.

NURSING IMPLICATIONS

Assessment

- Assess for infection (vital signs; appearance of wound, sputum, urine, and stool; WBC) at beginning of and throughout therapy.
- Obtain specimens for culture and sensitivity prior to therapy. First dose may be given before receiving results.
- Assess women of child bearing age for pregnancy. Women should have a negative serum pregnancy test before starting telavancin.
- Monitor bowel function. Diarrhea, abdominal cramping, fever, and bloody stools should be reported to health care professional promptly as a sign of pseudomembranous colitis. May begin up to several wks following cessation of therapy.
- Monitor for infusion reactions (Redman syndrome—flushing of upper body, urticaria, pruritus, rash). May resolve with stopping or slowing infusion.

- *Lab Test Considerations:* Monitor renal function (serum creatinine. creatinine clearance) prior to, every 48–72 hrs during, and at the end of therapy. May cause nephrotoxicity. If renal function ↓ s, reassess need for telavancin.
- May interfere with prothrombin time, INR, aPTT, activated clotting time, and coagulation based factor Xa tests. Collect blood samples for theses tests as close to next dose of telavancin as possible.
- Interferes with urine qualitative dipstick protein assays and quantitative dye methods; may use microalbumin assays.

Potential Nursing Diagnoses

Risk for infection (Indications)
Diarrhea (Adverse Reactions)

Implementation

IV Administration

- **Intermittent Infusion:** Reconstitute the 250 mg vial with 15 mL and the 750 mg vial with 45 mL of D5W, sterile water for injection, or 0.9% NaCl for concentrations of 15 mg/mL. Reconstitution time is usually under 2 min but may require up to 20 min. Mix thoroughly with contents dissolved completely. Do not administer solution that is discolored or contains particulate matter. Discard vial if vacuum did not pull diluent into vial. Time in vial plus time in bag should not exceed 4 hr at room temperature or 72 hr if refrigerated. *Diluent:* For doses of 150–800 mg dilute further with 100–250 mL of D5W, 0.9% NaCl, or LR. *Concentration:* For doses <150 mg or >800 mg dilute for a final concentration of 0.6–8 mg/mL. *Rate:* Administer over at least 60 min to minimize infusion reactions.
- **Y-Site Incompatibility:** Do not mix or administer with other medications. Flush line with D5W, 0.9% NaCl, or LR before and after administration.

Patient/Family Teaching

- Advise patient to take medication as directed, for full course of therapy, even if feeling well. If a dose is missed, contact health care professional promptly. Advise patient to read the *Medication Guide* before taking telavancin and with each Rx refill.

- Instruct patient to notify health care professional immediately if diarrhea, abdominal cramping, fever, or bloody stools occur and not to treat with antidiarrheals without consulting health care professionals.
- Inform patient that common side effects include taste disturbance, nausea, vomiting, headache and foamy urine. Notify health care professional if signs of infusion reaction occur.
- Advise patient to consult health care professional before taking other Rx, OTC, or herbal products.
- Advise female patients to use effective contraception during therapy and to notify health care professional if pregnancy is suspected. Encourage pregnant patients to enroll in the VIBATIV pregnancy registry by calling 1-888-658-4228.
- Instruct the patient to notify health care professional if symptoms do not improve.

Evaluation/Desired Outcomes

- Resolution of the signs and symptoms of infection. Length of time for complete resolution depends on the organism and site of infection.

tesamorelin
(tess-a-**moe**-rel-in)
Egrifta

Classification
Thera: none assigned
Pharm: growth hormone-releasing factor analogs

Pregnancy Category X

Indications
Reduction of excess abdominal fat (lipodystrophy) seen in HIV-infected patients.

Action
Acts as an analog of human growth hormone-releasing factor (GRF, GHRH), resulting in endogenous production of growth hormone (GH), which has anabolic and lipolytic properties. **Therapeutic Effects:** Reduction of abdominal adipose tissue in HIV-infected patients.

Pharmacokinetics
Absorption: <4% absorbed following subcutaneous administration.
Distribution: Unknown.
Metabolism and Excretion: Unknown.
Half-life: 26–38 min.

TIME/ACTION PROFILE (effect on visceral adipose tissue)

ROUTE	ONSET	PEAK	DURATION
Subcut	within 3 mos	10–12 mos	3 mos†

†Following discontinuation.

Contraindications/Precautions
Contraindicated in: Hypersensitivity to tesamorelin or mannitol; Any pathology that alters the hypothalamic-pituitary axis, including hypophysectomy, hypopituitarism, pituitary surgery/tumor, cranial irradiation/trauma; OB: may cause fetal harm; Lactation: Breastfeeding should be avoided by HIV-infected patients.

Use Cautiously in: Acute critical illness (may ↑ risk of serious complications; consider discontinuation); Pre-existing malignancy (disease should be inactive or treatment completed); Non-malignant neoplasms (carefully consider benefit); Persistently elevated Insulin-like Growth Factor (IGF-1; may require discontinuation); Diabetes mellitus (may cause glucose intolerance); Pedi: Safe and effective use in children not established.

Adverse Reactions/Side Effects
CV: peripheral edema. **Endo:** glucose intolerance. **Local:** erythema, hemorrhage, irritation, pain, pruritus. **MS:** arthralgia, carpal tunnel syndrome, extremity pain, myalgia. **Misc:** hypersensitivity reactions.

Interactions
Drug-Drug: May alter the clearance and actions of drugs known to be metabolized by the CYPP450 enzyme system including **corticosteroids, androgens, estro-**

gens and **progestins** (including **hormonal contraceptives**), **anticonvulsants**, and **cyclosporine**, careful monitoring for efficacy and/or toxicity recommended. Inhibits the conversion of **cortisone acetate** and **prednisone** to active forms; patients on replacement therapy may need ↑ maintenance/stress doses.

Route/Dosage
Subcut (Adults): 2 mg once daily.

Availability
Lyophilized powder for subcutaneous administration (requires reconstitution): 1 mg/vial.

NURSING IMPLICATIONS

Assessment
- Assess for fluid retention which manifests as ↑ tissue turgor and musculoskeletal discomfort (edema, arthralgia, extremity pain, carpal tunnel syndrome). May be transient or resolve with discontinuation of treatment.
- *Lab Test Considerations:* Monitor serum IGF-I closely during therapy; tesamorelin stimulates growth hormone production and the effect on progression of malignancies is unknown. Consider discontinuing tesamorelin in patients with persistent elevations of IGF-I levels, especially if efficacy response is not strong.
- May cause glucose intolerance and ↑ risk of developing diabetes. Monitor serum glucose prior to starting and periodically during therapy. Monitor diabetic patients closely for worsening of retinopathy.

Potential Nursing Diagnoses
Disturbed body image (Indications)

Implementation
- **Subcut:** Sterile Water for Injection 10 mL diluent is provided. Inject 2.2 mL of Sterile Water into tesamorelin, angled so that water goes down inside wall to prevent foaming. Roll vial gently between hands for 30 seconds to mix; do

not shake. Change needle. Withdraw solution and inject into 2nd tesamorelin vial with solution against wall of vial. Mix between hands for 30 seconds. Withdraw all solution (2 mg/2.2 mL). Solution is clear and colorless; do not administer solution that is discolored or contains particulate matter. Use solution immediately upon reconstitution or discard; do not refrigerate or freeze. Change needle to 1/2 inch 27 gauge needle. Pinch skin and inject at right angle into abdomen below navel; rotate sites. Remove hand from pinched area and inject slowly. Do not inject into scar, bruises, or the navel. Prior to reconstitution, vials must be refrigerated and protected from light.

Patient/Family Teaching
- Instruct patient on correct technique for administration of tesamorelin. Caution patient never to share needles with others.
- Inform patient that tesamorelin may cause symptoms of fluid retention (edema, arthralgia, carpal tunnel syndrome); usually transient or resolve with discontinuation of therapy.
- Advise patient to discontinue tesamorelin and notify health care professional promptly if signs and symptoms of hypersensitivity (rash, urticaria, hives, swelling of face or throat, shortness of breath, fast heartbeat, fainting) occur.
- Advise female patients to notify health care professional if pregnancy is planned or suspected or if breastfeeding.

Evaluation/Desired Outcomes
- Reduction of excess abdominal fat in HIV-infected patients with lipodystrophy.

☒ tetrabenazine
(te-tra-**ben**-a-zeen)
Xenazine

Classification
Thera: antichoreas
Pharm: reversible mono-
amine depleters

Pregnancy Category C

Indications

Treatment of chorea due to Huntington's Disease.

Action

Acts as a reversible inhibitor of the vesicle monoamine transporter type 2 (VMAT-2); which inhibits the reuptake of serotonin, norepinephrine and dopamine into vesicles in presynaptic neurons. **Therapeutic Effects:** ↓ chorea due to Huntington's Disease.

Pharmacokinetics

Absorption: At least 75% absorbed following oral administration.

Distribution: Crosses the blood-brain barrier.

Metabolism and Excretion: ⚠ Rapidly and extensively metabolized by the liver; CYP2D6 plays a large role in the metabolic process (the CYP2D6 enzyme system exhibits genetic polymorphism; ~7% of population may be poor metabolizers and may have significantly ↑ concentrations and an ↑ risk of adverse effects). Metabolites are renally excreted. Two metabolites α-dihydrotetrabenazine (α- HTBZ) and β-HTBZ bind to VMAT-2 and are pharmacologically active.

Half-life: α-HTBZ— 4-8 hrs; β-HTBZ—2-4 hr.

TIME/ACTION PROFILE (blood levels)

ROUTE	ONSET	PEAK	DURATION
PO	unknown	1.0–1.5 hr	12–18 hr*

*Return of symptoms following discontinuation.

Contraindications/Precautions

Contraindicated in: Hepatic impairment; Concurrent use of reserpine or MAO inhibitors; Patients who are actively suicidal or have untreated depression; Lactation: Lactation.

Use Cautiously in: History of/propensity for depression or history of psychiatric illness; history of suicidality; ⚠ Poor CYP2D6 metabolizers; initial dose reduction required; Concurrent use of CYP2D6 inhibitors; dose modification required; Recent history of myocardial infarction or unstable heart disease; OB: Use during pregnancy only when potential benefit justifies potential risk to the fetus; Pedi: Safety and efficacynot established.

Adverse Reactions/Side Effects

CNS: anxiety, <u>fatigue</u>, insomnia, depression, <u>sedation/somnolence</u>, cognitive defects, dizziness, headache. **Resp:** shortness of breath. **CV:** hypotension, QTc prolongation. **GI:** <u>nausea</u>, dysphagia. **Neuro:** <u>akathisia</u>, balance difficulty, dysarthria, parkinsonism, unsteady gait. **Misc:** NEUROLEPTIC MALIGNANT SYNDROME.

Interactions

Drug-Drug: Blood levels are ↑ by drugs that inhibit the CYP2D6 enzyme system including **fluoxetine**, **paroxetine**, and **quinidine**; initial dose reduction of tetrabenazine recommended. **Reserpine** binds to VMAT-2 and depletes monoamines in the CNS; avoid concurrent use; wait 3 wk after discontinuing to initiate tetrabenazine. Concurrent use of **MAO inhibitors** ↑ risk of serious adverse reactions and is contraindicated. Concurrent use with **neurolpetic drugs** or **dopamine antagonists** including **haloperidol**, **chlorpromazine**, **risperidone**, and **olanzapine** may ↑ risk of QTc prolongation, neuroleptic malignant syndrome and extrapyramidal disorders. Concurrent use of **alcohol** or other **CNS depressants** may ↑ risk of CNS depression.

Route/Dosage

⚠ **PO (Adults):** 12.5 mg/day for one wk initially, ↑ by 12.5 weekly up to 37.5–50 mg/day in three divided doses; *concurrent use of strong inhibitors or CYP2D6 or poor CYP2D6 metabolizers*— start with initial dose of 6.25 mg, titrate carefully.

Availability

Tablets: 12.5 mg, 25 mg.

NURSING IMPLICATIONS

Assessment

- Assess signs of Huntington's disease (changes in mood, cognition, chorea, rigidity, and functional capacity) periodically during therapy. Re-evaluate need for tetrabenazine periodically by assessing beneficial effect and side effects; determination may require dose reduction or discontinuation. Underlying chorea may improve over time, decreasing need for tetrabenazine.

- Monitor closely for new or worsening depression or suicidality. If depression or suicidality occurs ↓ dose and may initiate or ↑ dose of antidepressants.

- Monitor for signs of neuroleptic malignant syndrome (hyperpyrexia, muscle rigidity, altered mental status, irregular pulse or blood pressure, tachycardia, diaphoresis, cardiac dysrhythmia) periodically during therapy. If symptoms occur discontinue tetrabenazine and manage symptomatically. If re-introduction of tetrabenazine is considered monitor carefully; recurrences of neuroleptic malignant syndrome have occurred.

- Monitor patient for onset of akathisia (restlessness or desire to keep moving) and parkinsonian (difficulty speaking or swallowing, loss of balance control, pill rolling of hands, mask-like face, shuffling gait, rigidity, tremors). Notify health care professional if these symptoms occur; reduction in dose or discontinuation may be necessary.

- Assess blood pressure sitting and standing. May cause orthostatic hypotension.

- **Lab Test Considerations:** ⌘ Test for the CYP2D6 gene in patients requiring doses of >50 m g/day to determine if they are poor, intermediate, or extensive metabolizers. Limit dose to 50 mg in patients who are poor metabolizers.

Potential Nursing Diagnoses

Risk for suicide (Adverse Reactions)

Implementation

- Dose should be titrated slowly and individualized.
- **PO:** May be administered without regard to food.

Patient/Family Teaching

- Instruct patient to take tetrabenazine as directed. Do not take more or stop taking tetrabenazine without consulting health care professional. Dose adjustment may take several wk. Discuss procedure for missed doses with health care professional before beginning therapy; do not double doses. If a dose is missed or medication discontinued, involuntary movements will return or worsen in 12–18 hrs. If tetrabenazine is stopped for more than 5 days, consult health care professional before taking another dose; lower dose may be required.

- Advise patient and family to monitor for changes, especially sudden changes, in mood, behaviors, thoughts or feelings. If new or worse feelings of sadness or crying spells, lack of interest in friends or activities, sleeping a lot more or less, feelings of unimportance, guilt, hopelessness or helplessness, irritability or aggression, more or less hungry, difficulty paying attention, or thoughts of hurting self or ending life occur, notify health care professional promptly.

- Causes sedation. Caution patient to avoid driving and other activities requiring alertness until response to medication is known.

- Advise patient to avoid alcohol and other CNS depressants during therapy; ↑ s sedation.

- Inform patient of potential side effects and instruct to notify health care professional if side effects occur.

- Instruct patient to notify health care professional of all Rx or OTC medications, vitamins, or herbal products being taken and consult health care professional before taking any new medications.

✦ = Canadian drug name. ⌘ = Genetic implication.
*CAPITALS indicates life-threatening; underlines indicate most frequent.

- Advise female patients to notify health care professional if pregnancy is planned or suspected or if breastfeeding.

Evaluation/Desired Outcomes

- ↓ in chorea due to Huntington's disease.

---

tocilizumab
(toe-si-**liz**-oo-mab)
Actemra

Classification
Thera: antirheumatics, immunosuppressants
Pharm: interleukin antagonists

Pregnancy Category C

Indications

Treatment of adults with moderately- to severely-active rheumatoid arthritis who have not responded to one or more tumor necrosis factor (TNF) antagonist therapies. May be used alone or with methotrexate or other disease-modifying antirheumatic drugs (DMARDs).

Action

Acts as in inhibitor of interleukin-6 (IL-6) receptors by binding to them. IL-6 is a mediator of various inflammatory processes.
Therapeutic Effects: Slowed progression of rhuematoid arthritis.

Pharmacokinetics

Absorption: IV administration results in complete bioavailability.
Distribution: Unknown.
Metabolism and Excretion: Unknown.
Half-life: *4 mg/kg dose*—up to 11 days; *8 mg/kg*—up to 13 days.

TIME/ACTION PROFILE
(improvement)

ROUTE	ONSET	PEAK	DURATION
IV	within 1 mo	4 mos	unknown

Contraindications/Precautions

Contraindicated in: Serious infections; Patients at risk for GI perforation, including patients with diverticulitis; Active hepatic disease/impairment; Absolute neutrophil count (ANC) <2000/mm³ (<500/mm³ while on therapy) or platelet count below 100,000/mm³ (<50,000/mm³ while on therapy); Lactation: Not recommended during breastfeeding.
Use Cautiously in: Renal or hepatic impairment; Patients with tuberculosis risk factors; Geri: ↑ risk of adverse reactions; OB: Use during pregnancy only if potential benefit justifies potential risk to fetus; Pedi: Safe and effective use in children has not been established.

Adverse Reactions/Side Effects

CNS: headache, dizziness. **EENT:** nasopharyngitis. **Resp:** upper respiratory tract infections. **CV:** hypertension. **GI:** GASTROINTESTINAL PERFORATION, ↑ liver enzymes. **Derm:** rash. **Hemat:** NEUTROPENIA, THROMBOCYTOPENIA. **Metab:** ↑ lipids. **Misc:** serious infections including TUBERCULOSIS, DISSEMINATED FUNGAL INFECTIONS and INFECTIONS WITH OPPORTUNISTIC PATHOGENS, hypersensitivity reactions including ANAPHYLAXIS, infusion reactions.

Interactions

Drug-Drug: May alter the activity of CYP450 enzymes ; the effects of the following drugs should be monitored: **cycosporine**, **theophylline**, **warfarin**, **hormonal contraceptives**, **atorvastatin**, and **lovastatin**. Other drugs which are substrates for this system should also be monitored; effect may persist for several wks after discontinuation. May ↓ antibody response to and ↑ risk of adverse reactions to **live virus vaccines**; do not administer concurrently.

Route/Dosage

PO (Adults): 4 mg/kg may be ↑ to 8 mg/kg based on clinical response; dose reductions are recommended for elevated liver enzymes, neutropenia, and thrombocytopenia.

Availability

Solution for IV infusion (requires dilution): 20 mg/mL vial, 20 mg/4 mL vial, 200 mg/10 mL vial, 200 mg/20 mL vial and 400 mg/20 mL vial.

NURSING IMPLICATIONS

Assessment

- Assess pain and range of motion before and periodically during therapy.
- Assess for signs of infection (fever, dyspnea, flu-like symptoms, frequent or painful urination, redness or swelling at the site of a wound), including tuberculosis, prior to injection. Tocilizumab is contraindicated in patients with active infection. New infections should be monitored closely; most common are upper respiratory tract infections, bronchitis, and urinary tract infections. Signs and symptoms of inflammation may be lessened due to suppression from tocilizumab. Infections may be fatal, especially in patients taking immunosuppressive therapy. If patient develops a serious infection, discontinue tocilizumab until infection is controlled.
- Monitor for injection site reactions (redness and/or itching, rash, hemorrhage, bruising, pain, or swelling). Rash will usually disappear within a few days. Application of a towel soaked in cold water may relieve pain or swelling.
- Monitor patient for signs of anaphylaxis (urticaria, dyspnea, facial edema) following injection. Medications (antihistamines, corticosteroids, epinephrine) and equipment should be readily available in the event of a severe reaction. Discontinue tocilizumab immediately if anaphylaxis or other severe allergic reaction occurs.
- Assess patient for latent tuberculosis with a tuberculin skin test prior to initiation of therapy. Treatment of latent tuberculosis should be started before therapy with tocilizumab.
- Assess for signs and symptoms of systemic fungal infections (fever, malaise, weight loss, sweats, cough, dyspnea, pulmonary infiltrates, serious systemic illness with or without concomitant shock). Ascertain if patient lives in or has traveled to areas of endemic mycoses. Consider empiric antifungal treatment for patients at risk of histoplasmosis and other invasive fungal infections until the pathogens are identified. Consult with an infectious diseases specialist. Consider stopping tocilizumab until the infection has been diagnosed and adequately treated.
- **Lab Test Considerations:** Assess CBC with platelet count and liver function prior to initiating therapy and every 4–8 wks during therapy. Do not administer tocilizumab to patients with an absolute neutrophil count (ANC) <2000/ mm³, platelet count <100,000/mm³, or ALT or AST above 1.5 times the upper limit of normal (ULN).
- If ANC >1000/mm³, maintain dose. If ANC 500–1000/mm³, interrupt tocilizumab until ANC >1000/mm³, then resume at 4 mg/kg and ↑ to 8 mg/kg as clinically appropriate. If ANC <500/ mm³, discontinue tocilizumab.
- If platelet count 50,000–100,000/ mm³, interrupt dosing until platelet count is >100,000/mm³ then resume at 4 mg/kg and ↑ to 8 mg/kg as clinically appropriate. If platelet count is <50,000/mm³, discontinue tocilizumab.
- If liver enzymes persistently ↑ >1– 3x ULN, reduce tocilizumab dose to 4 mg/kg or interrupt until AST/ALT have normalized. If >3–5x ULN (confirmed by repeat testing), interrupt tocilizumab until <3x ULN and follow recommendations for ↑ >1–3x ULN. If >5x ULN, discontinue tocilizumab.
- Monitor lipid levels every 4–8 wks following initiation of therapy, then at 6 month intervals. May cause ↑ total cholesterol, triglycerides, LDL cholesterol, and/or HDL cholesterol.

Potential Nursing Diagnoses

Chronic pain (Indications)
Risk for infection (Adverse Reactions)

Implementation

- Administer a tuberculin skin test prior to administration of tocilizumab. Patients with latent TB should be treated for TB prior to therapy.

- Immunizations should be current prior to initiating therapy. Patients on tocilizumab may receive concurrent vaccinations, except for live vaccines.
- Do not administer solutions that are discolored or contain particulate matter. Discard unused solution.
- Other DMARDs should be continued during tocilizumab therapy.

IV Administration

- **Intermittent Infusion:** ***Diluent:*** Withdraw volume of 0.9% NaCl from a 100 mL bag equal to volume of solution required for patient's dose. Slowly add tocilizumab from each vial to infusion bag. Invert slowly to mix; avoid foaming. Do not infuse solutions that are discolored or contain particulate matter Diluted solution is stable for 24 hr if refrigerated or at room temperature; protect from light. Allow solution to reach room temperature before infusing. ***Rate:*** Infuse over 60 min. Do not administer via IV push or bolus.
- **Y-Site Incompatibility:** Do not infuse concomitantly in the same line with other drugs.

Patient/Family Teaching

- Instruct patient on the purpose for tocilizumab If a dose is missed, contact health care professional to schedule next infusion.
- Caution patient to notify health care professional immediately if signs of infection (fever, sweating, chills, muscle aches, cough, shortness of breath, blood in phlegm, weight loss, warm, red or painful skin or sores, diarrhea or stomach pain, burning on urination, urinary frequency, feeling tired), severe rash, swollen face, or difficulty breathing occurs while taking.
- Advise patient to consult health care professional before taking other Rx or OTC medications, vitamins, or herbal products.
- Instruct patient to notify health care professional of medication regimen prior to treatment or surgery.

- Advise female patients to notify health care professional if pregnancy is planned or suspected or if breastfeeding. Pregnant women should be encouraged to participate in the pregnancy registry by calling 1-877-311-8972.

Evaluation/Desired Outcomes

- ↓ pain and swelling with ↓ rate of joint destruction in patients with rheumatoid arthritis.

ulipristal (u-li-**priss**-tal)
Ella

Classification
Thera: contraceptive hormones (emergency)
Pharm: progesterone agonists/antagonists

Pregnancy Category X

Indications

Prevention of pregnancy following unprotected intercourse or known/suspected contraceptive failure; not intended for routine use.

Action

Binds to progesterone receptors. Delays follicular rupture, thereby inhibiting/delaying ovulation. Changes in endometrial environment may also contribute to action. **Therapeutic Effects:** Prevention of pregnancy.

Pharmacokinetics

Absorption: Well absorbed following oral administration.
Distribution: Unknown.
Protein Binding: >94%.
Metabolism and Excretion: Mostly metabolized by CYP3A4 enzyme system; one metabolite (monodemethyl-ulispristal) pharmacologically active.
Half-life: Uliprostal—32 hr; monodemethyl-ulispristal—27 hr.

TIME/ACTION PROFILE

ROUTE	ONSET	PEAK†	DURATION
PO	unknown	Ulipristal— 0.9 hr; monodeme- thyl-ulis- pristal—1 hr	unknown

†Blood level.

Contraindications/Precautions
Contraindicated in: Pregnancy or termination of existing pregnancy; Lactation: Not recommended during breastfeeding. **Use Cautiously in:** Repeated use; regular contraception should be continued/instituted and additional method should be used during current cycle.

Adverse Reactions/Side Effects
CNS: <u>headache</u>, dizziness, fatigue. **GI:** <u>abdominal pain</u>, <u>nausea</u>. **GU:** altered menstrual cycle, dysmenorrhea.

Interactions
Drug-Drug: Effectiveness may be ↓ by **drugs that induce the CYP3A4 enzyme system**, including **barbiturates**, **bosentan**, **carbamazepine**, **oxcarbazepine**, **phenytoin**, **topiramate**, **felbamate**, **griseofulvin**, **rifampin**. Effects may be ↑ **drugs that inhibit the CYP3A4 enzyme system** including **itraconazole** and **ketoconazole**. Efficacy of **hormonal contraceptives** may be ↓ during current cycle.
Drug-Natural Products: Effectiveness may be ↓ by **St. John's wort**.

Route/Dosage
PO (Adults): One tablet as soon as possible within 120 hours (5 days) after unprotected intercourse or known/suspected contraceptive failure. If vomiting occurs within 3 hrs dose may be repeated.

Availability
Tablet: 30 mg.

NURSING IMPLICATIONS

Assessment
- Exclude the possibility of pregnancy on the basis or history and/or physical exam or a pregnancy test before administering ulipristal.

Potential Nursing Diagnoses
Deficient knowledge, related to medication regimen (Patient/Family Teaching)

Implementation
- **PO:** Administer 1 tablet as soon as possible within 120 hrs (5 days) after unprotected intercourse or a known or suspected contraceptive failure. May be taken without regard to food. If vomiting occurs within 3 hrs of dose, may repeat. May be taken at any time during the menstrual cycle.
- Ulipristal may be less effective in women with a body mass index >30 k g/m².

Patient/Family Teaching
- Instruct patient to take ulipristal as directed. Advise patient that they should not take ulipristal if they know or suspect they are pregnant; ulipristal is not for use to end an existing pregnancy. Advise patient to contact health care professional if they vomit within 3 hrs after taking ulipristal.
- Inform patient that ulipristal may reduce the effectiveness of hormonal contraceptives. Advise patient to use a nonhormonal contraceptive during that menstrual cycle.
- Advise patient to notify health care professional and consider the possibility of pregnancy of their period is delayed by more than 1 wk beyond the expected date after taking ulipristal.
- Inform patient that ulipristal is not to be used as a routine form of contraception or to be used repeatedly within the same menstrual cycle.
- Advise patient that ulipristal does not protect against HIV infection and other sexually transmitted infections.
- Advise patient to notify health care professional if severe lower abdominal pain occurs 3–5 wks after taking ulipristal to be evaluated for an ectopic pregnancy.
- Instruct patient to notify health care professional of all Rx or OTC medica-

tions, vitamins, or herbal products being taken and consult health care professional before taking any new medications.

- Advise female patients to avoid breast-feeding if taking ulipristal.

Evaluation/Desired Outcomes
- Prevention of pregnancy.

---

velaglucerase alfa
(vel-a-gloo-ser-ase al-fa)
VPRIV

Classification
Thera: replacement enzyme (Gaucher's disease)
Pharm: enzymes

Pregnancy Category B

Indications
Enzyme replacement therapy (ERT) for pediatric and adult patients with type 1 Gaucher disease.

Action
Prevents the accumulation of glucocerebrosides in cells. Replaces glucocerebrosidases that are deficient in type 1 Gaucher's disease. Replaces the deficient enzyme in type 1 Gaucher disease. **Therapeutic Effects:** Improvement in symptoms of Gaucher's disease (anemia, thrombocytopenia, bone disease, splenomegaly, and hepatomegaly).

Pharmacokinetics
Absorption: IV administration results in complete bioavailability.
Distribution: Unknown.
Metabolism and Excretion: Unknown.
Half-life: 11–12 min.

TIME/ACTION PROFILE

ROUTE	ONSET	PEAK	DURATION
IV	unknown	unknown	unknown

Contraindications/Precautions
Contraindicated in: None noted.
Use Cautiously in: Previous hypersensitivity reactions; pretreament required; Geri: consider concurrent disease states

and drug therapy; OB: Use during pregnancy only if clearly needed; Lactation: Use catiously if breast-feeding; Pedi: Safe and effective use in children <4 yr not established.

Adverse Reactions/Side Effects
CNS: dizziness, fatigue, headache, <u>weakness</u>. **CV:** hypertension, hypotension. **GI:** <u>abdominal pain</u>, nausea. **Derm:** rash (↑ in children), flushing, urticaria. **Hemat:** <u>↑ aPTT(↑ in children)</u>. **MS:** back pain, <u>joint pain</u>, bone pain. **Misc:** hypersensitivity reactions including ANAPHYLAXIS, fever (↑ in children), <u>infusion-related reactions</u>.

Interactions
Drug-Drug: None noted.

Route/Dosage
PO (Adults): 60 Units/kg every other week.

Availability
Lyophilized powder for IV injection (requires reconstitution and dilution): 200 Units/vial, 400 Units/vial.

NURSING IMPLICATIONS

Assessment
- Monitor for an improvement in symptoms including hepatomegaly, splenomegaly, anemia, thrombocytopenia, bone demineralization, and ↑ appetite and energy level periodically during therapy.
- Monitor patient for signs of hypersensitivity reactions (pruritus, flushing, urticaria, angioedema, chest pain, dyspnea, hypotension). Pretreatment with antihistamines and decreasing rate of infusion usually allows patient to continue use.
- Monitor for signs and symptoms of infusion-related reactions (headache, dizziness, hypotension, hypertension, nausea, fatigue, pyrexia). Most reactions are mild, occur within the 1st 6 months of therapy, and diminish with time. May be treated with slowing infusion rate, antihistamines, antipyretics, corticosteroids, and/or stopping infusion and resuming with ↑ infusion time.

- *Lab Test Considerations:* Monitor hemoglobin and platelet count monthly to determine effectiveness of therapy.
- May cause prolonged activated partial thromboplastin time.

Potential Nursing Diagnoses
Fatigue (Indications)
Risk for injury (Indications)

Implementation
- Patients currently treated with imiglucerase may switch to velaglucerase. If on a stable imiglucerase dose, begin treatment with velaglucerase at the same dose.
- Pre-treatment with antihistamines, and/or corticosteroids may prevent subsequent infusion-related reactions.
- Determine correct amount of velaglucerase and appropriate number of vials. Reconstitute each 200 unit vial with 2.2 mL and each 400 unit vial with 4.3 mL of Sterile Water for Injection. Mix vials gently; do not shake. Solution is clear to slightly opalescent and colorless; do not administer solutions that are discolored or contain particulate matter. *Concentration:* 100 Units/mL. Withdraw 2 mL from each 200 Unit vial and 4 mL from each 400 Unit vial. *Diluent:* Dilute total volume in 100 mL of 0.9% NaCl. Administer within 24 hrs of reconstitution. Do not freeze; protect from light. *Rate:* Infuse diluted solution over 1 hr through an in-line low protein-binding 0.2 mcg filter.
- **Additive Incompatibility:** Do not infuse with other solutions or products.

Patient/Family Teaching
- Inform patient of the purpose of this medication and the importance of treatment at least every 4 wk. Velaglucerase helps control the symptoms but does not cure Gaucher's disease. Lifelong therapy may be required.
- Advise female patient to notify health care professional if pregnancy is planned or suspected or if breastfeeding.
- Emphasize the importance of follow-up examinations and lab tests.

Evaluation/Desired Outcomes
- Increasing hemoglobin and platelet counts and decreasing acid phosphatase levels, hepatomegaly, and splenomegaly. In pediatric patients, cachexia and wasting should diminish.

vigabatrin
(vye-**gah**-bat-rin)
Sabril

Classification
Thera: anticonvulsants

Pregnancy Category C

Indications
Management (adjunctive) of refractory Complex Partial Seizures in Adults in patients who have responded inadequately to several alternative treatments; not a first-line treatment. Management of infantile spasms (IS) in patients 1 mo – 2 yr.

Action
Acts an irreversible inhibitor of γ-aminobutyric acid transaminase (GABA-T), the enzyme responsible for the metabolism of the inhibitory neurotransmitter GABA. This action results in ↑ levels of GABA in the central nervous system. **Therapeutic Effects:** ↓ incidence and severity of refractory Complex Partial Seizures.

Pharmacokinetics
Absorption: Completely absorbed following oral administration.
Distribution: Enters breast milk, remainder of distribution unknown.
Metabolism and Excretion: Minimal metabolism, mostly eliminated unchanged in urine.
Half-life: 7.5 hr.

TIME/ACTION PROFILE
(anticonvulsant effect)

ROUTE	ONSET	PEAK	DURATION
PO	unknown	1 hr†	12 hr‡

†Blood level.

‡Clinical benefit should be seen in 2 – 4 wk for IS or within 3 mo for complex partial seizures.

Contraindications/Precautions

Contraindicated in: History or high risk of other types of irreversible vision loss unless benefits of treatment clearly outweigh risks; OB: Use during pregnancy only if the potential benefit justifies the potential risk to the fetus (may cause fetal harm); Lactation: Enters breast milk; breastfeeding should be avoided.

Use Cautiously in: Renal impairment (dose modification recommended for CCr <50 mL/min); History of suicidal ideation; Geri: Consider age-related ↓ in renal function adjust dose accordingly (↑ risk of sedation/confusion); Pedi: abnormal MRI signal changes have been seen in infants.

Adverse Reactions/Side Effects

CNS: SUICIDAL THOUGHTS, confusional state, memory impairment, drowsiness, fatigue. **CV:** edema. **EENT:** blurred vision, nystagmus, vision loss. **Hemat:** anemia. **Metab:** weight gain. **MS:** arthralgia. **Neuro:** abnormal coordination, tremor, peripheral neuropathy.

Interactions

Drug-Drug: Should not be used concurrently with other **drugs having adverse ocular effects**; ↑ risk of additive toxicity. May ↓ **phenytoin** levels and effectiveness.

Route/Dosage

PO (Adults): 500 mg twice daily initially, may be ↑ in 500 mg increments every 7 days depending on response up to 1.5 g twice daily.

Renal Impairment

PO (Adults): *CCr >50–80 mL/min—* ↓ dose by 25%; *CCr >30–50 mL/min—* ↓ dose by 50%; *CCr >10–<30 mL/min—* ↓ dose by 75%.

PO (Children 1 mo–2 yr): 50 mg/kg/day given in 2 divided doses initially, increasing by 25-50 mg/kg/day increments every 3 days up to a maximum of 150 mg/kg/day; dosage adjustments are necessary for renal impairment.

Availability

Tablets: 500 mg. **Powder packets for oral solution:** 500 mg/packet.

NURSING IMPLICATIONS

Assessment

- Assess location, duration, and characteristics of seizure activity. Institute seizure precautions. Assess response to and continued need for vigabatrin periodically during therapy.
- Monitor closely for notable changes in behavior that could indicate the emergence or worsening of suicidal thoughts or behavior or depression.
- Test vision at baseline (no later than 4 wks after starting), at least every 3 months during, and 3–6 months after discontinuation of therapy.
- Assess for signs and symptoms of peripheral neuropathy (numbness or tingling or toes or feet, reduced lower limb vibration or position sensation, progressive loss of reflexes, starting at ankles).
- **Lab Test Considerations:** Monitor CBC periodically during therapy. May cause anemia.
- May cause ↓ AST and ALT levels precluding use to detect hepatic injury.
- May ↑ amino acids in urine causing false positive results of genetic metabolic diseases.

Potential Nursing Diagnoses

Risk for injury (Indications)
Disturbed sensory perception (Adverse Reactions)

Implementation

- Available only through SHARE program of restricted distribution. Only prescribers and pharmacies registered in the program and patients enrolled in the program have access. Contact SHARE program at 1-888-45-SHARE.
- **PO:** Administer twice daily without regard to food.
- Mix oral solution for babies by mixing the powder in each packet with 10 mL of water; may be cold or room temperature. Follow manufacturer's instruction for mixing oral solution. Oral solution may be administered at the same time as food, but should only be mixed with water.

Patient/Family Teaching

- Enroll patient in SHARE Program. Instruct patient to take vigabatrin around the clock, as directed. Medication should be gradually discontinued to prevent seizures. Advise patient to read the *Medication Guide* before starting therapy and with each Rx refill.
- Educate patient on risks of vigabatrin. Inform patient of the risk of permanent vision loss, particularly loss of peripheral vision, and that vision loss may not be detected before it is severe and is irreversible. Emphasize the importance of monitoring vision every 3 months. Advise patient to notify health care professional immediately if changes in vision are suspected.
- May cause drowsiness, ataxia, fatigue and confusion. Caution patient to avoid driving or other activities requiring alertness until response to medication is known. Tell patient not to resume driving until physician gives clearance based on control of seizure disorder.
- Inform patients and families of risk of suicidal thoughts and behavior and advise that behavioral changes, emergency or worsening signs and symptoms of depression, unusual changes in mood, or emergence of suicidal thoughts, behavior, or thoughts of self-harm should be reported to health care professional immediately.
- Advise patient to notify health care professional if an ↑ in seizures, weight gain, or edema occurs or if sleepiness, ear infection, or irritability occurs in an infant.
- Advise patient to consult health care professional before taking other Rx, OTC, or herbal preparation and to avoid taking alcohol or other CNS depressants concurrently with lacosamide.
- Advise female patients to notify health care professional if pregnancy is planned or suspected or if breast feeding. Encourage pregnant patients to enroll in the North American Antiepileptic Drug (NAAED) Pregnancy Registry by calling 1-888-233-2334; information is available at www.aedpregnancyregistry.org.

Evaluation/Desired Outcomes

- ↓ seizure activity. If no substantial clinical benefit within 3 months of initiation, discontinue vigabatrin.
- ↓ in infantile spasms. If no substantial clinical benefit within 2–4 wk of initiation, discontinue vigabatrin.

vilazodone
(vil-**az**-oh-done)
Viibryd

Classification
Thera: antidepressants
Pharm: selective norepinephrine reuptake inhibitors, benzofurans

Pregnancy Category C

Indications
Treatment of major depressive disorder.

Action
↑ s serotonin activity in the CNS by inhibiting serotonin reuptake. **Therapeutic Effects:** Improvement in symptoms of depression.

Pharmacokinetics
Absorption: 72% absorbed following oral administration with food.
Distribution: Unknown.
Protein Binding: 96–99%.
Metabolism and Excretion: Mostly metabolized by the liver, primarily by the CYP3A4 enzyme system; 1% excreted unchanged in urine.
Half-life: 25 hr.

TIME/ACTION PROFILE (blood levels)

ROUTE	ONSET	PEAK	DURATION
PO	unknown	4–5 hr	unknown

Contraindications/Precautions

Contraindicated in: Concurrent use or within 14 days of starting or stopping MOAIs; Severe hepatic impairment.

Use Cautiously in: History of seizure disorder; History of suicide attempt/suicidal ideation; Bipolar disorder; may ↑ risk of mania/hypomania; OB: Use during pregnancy only if maternal benefit outweighs fetal risk; use during third trimester may result in need for prolonged hospitalization, respiratory support and tube feeding; Lactation: Breast feed only if maternal benefit outweighs newborn risk; Pedi: Safe and effective use in children not established; ↑ risk of suicidal thinking/behavior in children, adolescents, and young adults.

Adverse Reactions/Side Effects

CNS: NEUROLEPTIC MALIGNANT-LIKE SYNDROME, SEIZURES, SUICIDAL THOUGHTS, insomnia, abnormal dreams, dizziness. **GI:** diarrhea, nausea, dry mouth, restlessness, vomiting. **Endo:** ↓ libido, sexual dysfunction, syndrome of inappropriate antidiuretic hormone (SIADH). **F and E:** hyponatremia. **Hemat:** bleeding. **Misc:** SEROTONIN SYNDROME.

Interactions

Drug-Drug: Concurrent use with, or use within 14 days of starting or stopping **MAOIs** may ↑ risk of neuroleptic malignant syndrome or serotonin syndrome and should be avoided. Concurrent use with **NSAIDs**, **aspirin**, **antiplatelet drugs**, or other **drugs that affect coagulation** may ↑ risk of bleeding. Concurrent use of **strong inhibitors of CYP3A4**, including **ketoconazole** ↑ blood levels and the risk of adverse reactions/toxicity; daily dose should not exceed 20 mg. Concurrent use of **moderate inhibitors of CYP3A4**, including **erythromycin** may require dose reduction to 20 mg daily if adverse reactions/toxicity occurs. Concurrent use with other **drugs that alter CNS serotonergic neurotransmitters** including **SSRIs**, **SNRIs**, **triptans**, **buspirone**, **tramadol**, and **typtophan products** may ↑ risk of serotonin syndrome and should be under-

taken with caution. Use cautiously with other **CNS-active drugs**.

Route/Dosage

PO (Adults): 10 mg once daily for one week, then 20 mg once daily for one week, then 40 mg once daily. *Concurrent use of strong inhibitors of CYP3A4—daily dose should not exceed 20 mg.*

Availability

Tablets: 10 mg, 20 mg, 40 mg.

NURSING IMPLICATIONS

Assessment

- Assess mental status and mood changes. Inform health care professional if patient demonstrates significant ↑ in anxiety, nervousness, or insomnia.
- Prior to starting therapy, screen patient for bipolar disorder (detailed psychiatric history, including family history of suicide, bipolar disorder, depression). Use cautiously in patients with a positive history.
- Assess suicidal tendencies, especially in early therapy. Restrict amount of drug available to patient. Risk may be ↑ in children, adolescents, and adults ≤24 yr.
- Assess for signs and symptoms of hyponatremia (headache, difficulty concentrating, memory impairment, confusion, weakness, unsteadiness). May require discontinuation of therapy.
- Assess for serotonin syndrome (mental changes [agitation, hallucinations, coma], autonomic instability [tachycardia, labile blood pressure, hyperthermia], neuromuscular aberrations [hyper-reflexia, incoordination], and/or GI symptoms [nausea, vomiting, diarrhea]), especially in patients taking other serotonergic drugs (SSRIs, SNRIs, triptans).
- Monitor for development of neuroleptic malignant syndrome (fever, muscle rigidity, altered mental status, respiratory distress, tachycardia, seizures, diaphoresis, hypertension or hypotension, pallor, tiredness, loss of bladder control). Discontinue vilazodone and notify health care professional immediately if these symptoms occur.

- *Lab Test Considerations:* Monitor serum sodium concentrations periodically during therapy. May cause hyponatremia potentially as a result of syndrome of inappropriate antidiuretic hormone secretion (SIADH).
- May cause altered anticoagulant effects. Monitor patients receiving warfarin, NSAIDs, or aspirin concurrently.

Potential Nursing Diagnoses

Ineffective coping (Indications)
Risk for injury (Side Effects)

Implementation

- **PO:** Administer vilazodone with food; administration without food can result in inadequate drug concentrations and may ↓ effectiveness.

Patient/Family Teaching

- Instruct patient to take vilazodone as directed at the same time each day. Take missed doses as soon as possible unless almost time for next dose. Do not double doses or discontinue abruptly. Gradually ↓ dose before discontinuation. Advise patient to read *Medication Guide* before starting therapy and with each Rx refill; new information may be available.
- Advise patient, family, and caregivers to look for activation of mania/hypomania and suicidality, especially during early therapy or dose changes. Notify health care professional immediately if thoughts about suicide or dying, attempts to commit suicide; new or worse depression or anxiety; agitation or restlessness; panic attacks; insomnia; new or worse irritability; aggressiveness; acting on dangerous impulses, mania, or other changes in mood or behavior or if symptoms of serotonin syndrome occur.
- Caution patient of the risk or serotonin syndrome and neuroleptic malignant syndrome, especially when taking triptans, tramadol, tryptophan supplements and other serotonergic or antipsychotic agents.
- May cause dizziness. Caution patient to avoid driving or other activities requiring alertness until response to the drug is known.
- Instruct patient to notify health care professional of all Rx or OTC medications, vitamins, or herbal products being taken and to avoid concurrent use of Rx, OTC, and herbal products, especially NSAIDs, aspirin, and warfarin, without consulting health care professional.
- Caution patient to avoid taking alcohol or other CNS-depressant drugs during therapy.
- Instruct female patients to inform health care professional if pregnancy is planned or suspected or if breastfeeding.
- Emphasize the importance of follow-up exams to monitor progress. Encourage patient participation in psychotherapy.

Evaluation/Desired Outcomes

- ↑ sense of well-being.
- Renewed interest in surroundings. Need for therapy should be periodically reassessed. Therapy is usually continued for several months.
- ↓ anxiety.

Table 1 Drugs With New Warnings

Generic name (Brand name)	Warning
acetaminophen	Prescription combinations containing acetaminophen will be limited to 325 mg/tablet or capsule. Warning strengthened about risk of liver injury with daily doses >4000 mg or concurrent use of alcohol.
Antipsychotics including aripiprazole (Abilify), asenapine (Saphris), chlorpromazine (Thorazine), clozapine (Clozaril), haloperidol (Haldol), iloperidone (Fanapt), loxapine (Loxitane), olanzapine (Zyprexa), olanzapine/fluoxetine (Symbyax), molindone (Moban), paliperidone (Invega), pimozide (Orap), quetiapine (Seroquel), risperidone (Risperdal), thiothixene (Navane), trifluoperazine (Stelazine), ziprasidone (Geodon, Fazaclo)	Class labeling change: Potential risk for abnormal muscle movements (including EPS) and withdrawal symptoms in newborns whose mothers received them during the third trimester Symptoms may include agitation, abnormally ↑ or ↓ muscle tone, tremor, drowsiness, severe difficulty breathing, difficulty feeding, may subside within hrs or days and may not require treatment. Medications in mother should not be discontinued without consulting health care professional.
benzonatate (Tessalon)	Accidental ingestion resulting in overdose by children <10 yr can result in serious side effects including cardiac arrest, coma, seizures and death. Children may be attracted by the candy-like appearance (a round, liquid-filled gelatin capsule).
bevacizumab (Avastin)	Breast cancer indication removed, not found to be safe and effective.
Biphosphonates including alendronate (Fosamax), etidronate (Didronel, ✽ Didrocal), ibandronate (Boniva), pamidronate (Aredia), risedronate (Actonel), tiludronate (Skelid), zoledronic acid (Reclast, Zometa)	↑ risk of atypical femur fractures.
clopidogrel (Plavix)	Reduced effectiveness in poor metabolizers may lead to serious thrombotic events; effectiveness may also be reduced by concurrent use of omeprazole and should be avoided.
deferasirox (Exjade)	May cause potentially fatal renal/hepatic toxicity or GI bleeding.
dolasetron (Anzemet)	High IV dose for nausea and vomiting due to chemotherapy is no longer recommended due to risk of arrhythmias.
erythromycin (E-Mycin, EES, Erythrocin)	↑ blood levels and risk of serious toxicity when used with ergotamine, dihydroergotamine, or colchicine; concurrent use should be avoided.
estrogenspray (Estramist)	↑ risk of estrogenic effects in inadvertently exposed children or pets.

Table 1 (Continued)

FLUOROQUINOLONES including ciprofloxacin (Cipro, Proquin), gemifloxacin (Factive), levofloxacin (Levaquin), moxifloxacin (Avelox), norfloxacin (Noroxin), ofloxacin (Floxin)	Risk of exacerbating muscle weakness in patients with myasthenia gravis. fluoroquinolones should be avoided in patients with a known history of myasthenia gravis.
GnRH agonists including goserelin (Zoladex), histrelin (Vantas), leuprolide (Eligard, Lupron, Viadur), nafarelin (Synarel), triptorelin (Trelstar)	↑ risk of diabetes mellitus and adverse cardiovascular reactions.
lamotrigine (Lamictal)	May cause aseptic meningitis.
Long-acting beta-agonists (LABAs) including formoterol (Foradil), salmeterol (Serevent)	New labeling: contraindicated without an asthma controller medication such as inhaled corticosteroid, single-agents should only be used in combination with an asthma controller medication; should only be used long-term when asthma cannot be adequately controlled on controller medications and then for shortest duration possible. Maintenance therapy should be an asthma controller medication. Children and adolescents requiring LABAs in addition to an inhaled corticosteroid should use combination products to ensure compliance.
lopinavir/ritonaviroral solution (Kaletra)	Risk of serious adverse reactions due to presence of alcohol and propylene glycol in the oral solution may result in serious heart, kidney, or breathing problems in babies <14 days old; use should be avoided in premature babies until 14 days after their due date, or in full-term babies younger than 14 days of age unless benefit outweighs potential risks.
olanzapine (Zyprexa)	Clinicians should consider the ↑ potential and long-term risks for weight gain and hyperlipidemia. Available alternative treatments should be considered in this age group.
orlistat (Alli/Xenical)	May rarely result in severe liver injury.
Proton-Pump Inhibitors including esopmeprazole magnesium (Nexium), esomeprazole magnesium/naproxen (Vimovo), dexlansoprazole (Dexilant), omeprazole (Prilosec/Prilosec OTC), omeprazole/sodium bicarbonate (Zegerid/Zegerid OTC), lansoprazole (Prevacid/Prevacid 24 HR), pantoprazole sodium (Protonix), rabeprazole sodium (AcipHex)	Prolonged (>1 yr) use may result in potentially serious hypomagnesemia which can cause serious adverse events (including muscle spasm, arrhythmias and seizures). Magnesium supplementation alone may not improve low serum magnesium levels. May ↑ risk of fractures of hip, wrist, and spine.

Table 1 Drugs With New Warnings (Continued)

quinine (Quilaquin)	Serious life-threatening hematologic reactions including thrombocytopenia, hemolytic uremic syndrome/thrombotic thrombocytopenic purpura in addition to hypersensitivity reactions and serious arrythmias; only approved indication is malaria, not be used in the treatment/prevention of nocturnal leg cramps.
rosiglitazone (Avandia)	Due to ↑ risk of adverse cardiovascular events, use should be limited to those who have not responded to safer medications for type 2 diabetes.
saquinavir (Invirase)	↑ risk of arrhythmias.
terbutaline (Bricanyl)	Injectable terbutaline should not be used in pregnant women for prevention or prolonged treatment (beyond 72 hrs) of preterm labor due to potential for serious maternal heart problems and death. Oral terbutaline should not be used for prevention/treatment of preterm labor.
topiramate (Topamax)	↑ risk of cleft lip/palate in infants born to mothers who take topiramate during pregnancy; pregnancy category changed to "D."
tramadol (Ultram)	↑ suicide risk in patients with history of substance abuse/addiction, concurrent use of sedative hypnotics or antidepressants.

Table 2 Drugs with New Dosage Forms or Strengths

Generic name (Brand name)	New dosage form or strength
adapalene (Differin)	Lotion 0.1% formulation for acne.
aztreonam (Cayston)	Inhalation solution 75 mg/vial.
buprenorphine (Butrans)	Transdermal opioid agonist/antagonist analgesic patch (5 mcg/hr, 10 mcg/hr, 20 mcg/hr) for moderate to severe pain.
calcipotriene (Sorilux)	Foam formulation 0.005% for plaque psoriasis.
cetirizine (Zyrtec)	Orally-disintegrating tablets 10 mg for relief of allergy symptoms.
clonidine (Kapvay)	Extended-release tablets 0.1 mg, 0.2 mg for the management of ADHD.
doxepin (Silenor)	Tablets 3 mg and 6 mg for insomnia.
ethinyl estradiol/norethindrone/iron (Femcon Fe)	Chewable spearmint-flavored tablets ethinyl estradiol 0.035 mg/norethindrone 0.4 mg (iron is not therapeutic) for hormonal contraception.
gabapentin (Gralise)	Extended—release tablets 300 mg and 600 mg for once daily treatment of post-herpetic neuralgia.
gatifloxacin (Zymaxid)	Ophthalmic solution 0.5% for bacterial conjunctivitis.
glycopyrrolate (Cuvposa)	Oral solution 1 mg/5 mL for management of chronic drooling in children 3 – 16 yr with neurologic disorders.
hydromorphone (Exalgo)	Oral extended release tablets 8, 12 and 16 mg for moderate to severe chronic pain.
ketorolac (Sprix)	Nasal spray 15.75 mg/spray for moderate to moderately severe pain.
lacosamide (Vimpat)	Oral solution 10 mg/mL for partial-onset seizures.
mannitol (Aridol)	Inhalation formulation in 40 mg/cap for administration in graduated doses to assess bronchial responsiveness.
memantine (Namenda XR)	Extended release capsule 7 mg, 14, mg, 21 mg and 28 mg for Alzheimer's disease.
moxifloxacin (Moxeza)	Ophthalmic solution 0.5% for bacterial conjuctivitis.
ondansetron (Zuplenz)	Oral soluble film 4 mg and 8 mg for prevention of nausea and vomiting.
pramipexole (Mirapex ER)	Extended—release tablet 0.375 mg, 0.75 mg, 1.5 mg, 3 mg, 4.5 mg for Parkinson's disease.

Table 2 (Continued)

pregabalin (Lyrica)	Oral solution 20 mg/mL for various pain-related syndromes.
risedronate (Atelvia)	35 mg delayed-release once-weekly phosphonate tablets for osteoporosis can be taken after breakfast.
rufinamide (Banzel)	Oral Suspension, 40 mg/mL for adjunctive treatment of seizures associated with Lennox-Gastaut syndrome.
testosterone (Axiron)	Topical solution (30 mg/pump) for underarm application for replacement therapy.
testosterone (Fortesta)	Topical gel formulation 10 mg/5 gm activation (thigh application) for replacement therapy.
pneumococcal vaccine, 13-valent conjugate [PCV13] (Prevnar)	Expanded from PCV7 vaccine to include more serotypes, will replace PCV7 to prevent pneumococcal disease in infants and children <6 yr.
trazodone (Oleptro)	Extended-release tablets 150 mg and 300 mg for treatment of depression.
miconazole (Oravig)	Buccal tablet 50 mg for treatment of oropharyngeal candidiasis.
vardenafil (Staxyn	Orally-disintegrating tablet 10 mg for erectile dysfunction.

Table 3 Drugs with New Indications

Generic name (Brand name)	New indication
aripiprazole (Abilify)	Treatment of irritability associated with autistic disorder.
atazanavir (Reyataz)	Treatment of HIV during pregnancy and postpartum period.
denosumab (Xgeva)	Prevention of skeletal-related events, including pathological fractures, spinal cord compression or radiation to bone, caused by bone metastases from solid tumors (also marketed as Prolia for treatment of post-menopausal osteoporosis).
duloxetine (Cymbalta)	Chronic musculoskeletal pain including osteoarthritis and low back pain.
human papillomavirus vaccine, recombinant (Gardasil)	Prevention of anal cancer and associated lesions in people ages 9–26 yr.
Meningococcal [Groups A, C, Y and W-135] Oligosaccharide Diphtheria CRM197 Conjugate Vaccine (Menveo)	Active immunization to prevent invasive meningococcal disease in children 2–10 yr.
onabotulinumtoxinA (Botox)	Treatment of chronic migraine.

Table 4 New Drug Combinations

Brand name	Components, dosages, and indications
Amturnide	aliskiren 150 mg + amlopidine 5 mg + hydrochlorothiazide 12.5 mg aliskiren 300 mg + amlopidine 5 mg + hydrochlorothiazide 12. 5 mg aliskiren 300 mg + amlopidine 5 mg + hydrochlorothiazide 25 mg aliskiren 300 mg + amlopidine 10 mg + hydrochlorothiazide 12.5 mg aliskiren 300 mg + amlopidine 10mg + hydrochlorothiazide 12.5 mg renin inhibitor/calcium channel blocker/diuretic for the treatment of hypertension.
Beyaz	drospirenone 3 mg + ethinyl estradiol 0.02 mg + levomefolate 0.451 mg Hormonal oral contraceptive containing folate.
Jalyn	dutasteride 0.5 mg + tamsulosin 0.4 mg 5-alpha-reductase inhibitor alpha blocker for treatment of BPH.
Dulera	formoterol 0.005 mg + mometasone 0.1 mg + formoterol 0.005 mg + mometasone 0.2mg long acting beta-agonist/corticosteroid for maintenance treatment of asthma.
Kobiglyze XR	metformin 500 mg + saxagliptin 5 mg metformin 1000 mg + saxagliptin 5 mg metformin 1000 mg + saxagliptin 2.5 mg biguanide/dipeptidyl peptidase-4 inhibitor for Type 2 Diabetes.
Lo Loestrin FE	24 tablets of ethinyl estradiol 10 mcg + norethindrone acetate 1 mg 2 tablets of ethinyl estradiol 10 mcg 2 tablets of ferrous fumarate 75 mg Very low dose hormonal contraceptive plus iron.
Malarone	*Adult tablets* — atovaquone 250 mg + proguanil 100 mg *Pediatric tablets* — atovaquone 62.5 mg + proguanil 25 mg For the prevention and treatment of malaria.
Nuedexta	dextromethorphan 20 mg + quinidine 10 mg Cough suppressant/enzyme inhibitor for Pseudobulbar affect.

Table 4 (Continued)

Satyral	drospirenone 3 mg + ethinyl estradiol 0.03 mg + levomefolate 0.451 Hormonal contraceptive plus folate.
Suprep	magnesium sulfate 1.6 gm per bottle + potassium sulfate 3.13 gm per bottle + sodium sulfate 17. 5 gm Osmotic laxative for colon cleansing in preparation for colonoscopy in adults.
Tekamlo	aliskiren 150 mg + amlodipine 5 mg aliskiren 150 mg + amlodipine 10 mg aliskiren 300 mg + amlodipine 5 mg aliskiren 300 mg + amlodipine 10 mg Combination renin inhibitor and calcium channel blocker for hypertension.
Tribenzor	olmesartan 20 mg + amlodipine 5 mg + hydrochlorothiazide 12.5 mg olmesartan 40 mg + amlodipine 5 m g + hydrochlorothiazide 12.5 mg olmesartan 40 mg + amlodipine 5 mg + hydrochlorothiazide 25 mg olmesartan 40 mg + amlodipine 10 mg + hydrochlorothiazide 12.5 mg olmesartan 40 mg + amlodipine 10 mg + hydrochlorothiazide 25 mg
Veltin	*Topical gel* — clindamycin 1.2% + tretinoin 0.025% For the topical treatment of acne vulgaris in patients >12 yr.
Vimovo	esomeprazole 20 mg + naproxen 375 mg and esomeprazole 20 mg + naproxen 500 mg Delayed-release tablets for arthritis patients at risk for NSAID-associated gastric ulcers.

Table 5 Discontinued Drugs

Generic name (Brand name)	Reason for discontinuation
gemtuzumab ozogamicin (Mylotarg)	Safety concerns and lack of clinical benefit.
sibutramine (Meridia)	↑ Risk of serious cardiovascular effects (heart attack, stroke).
propoxyphene (Darvocet, Darvon)	↑ Risk of serious and potentially fatal arrhythmias.

Where's the SECRET CODE?

It's inside your copy of

DAVIS'S DRUG GUIDE for NURSES®, TWELFTH EDIT
or
NURSE'S MED DECK, TWELFTH EDITION

Davis's Drug Guide Online
powered by Unbound Medicine®

Activate your FREE, 1-year subscription!

✓ Access the complete
Davis's Drug Guide for Nurses
database—over 1,100 monographs
in all—from your desktop, laptop,
or any mobile device with a web browser.

FREE mobile download!

✓ Download monographs for 100 top drug
to your mobile device for quick reference
anytime, anywhere.

If you've bought the version of Davis's
Drug Guide for Nurses or Med Deck w
the Resource Kit CD-ROM, follow the
on the CD–or–simply type the following
address into your web browser:
www.drugguide.com/ddo/ub/bookcode

Download your FREE monographs!

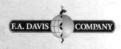
F.A. DAVIS COMPANY

www.FADavis.com